# Alternating Electric Fields Therapy in Oncology

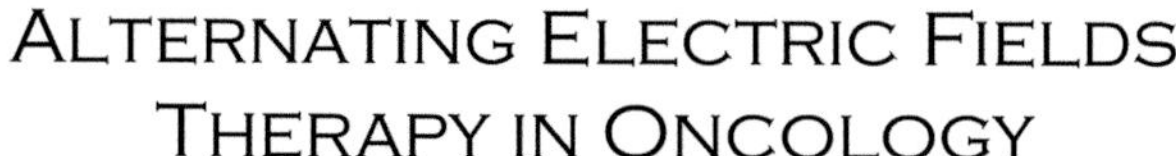

# Alternating Electric Fields Therapy in Oncology

## A Practical Guide to Clinical Applications of Tumor Treating Fields

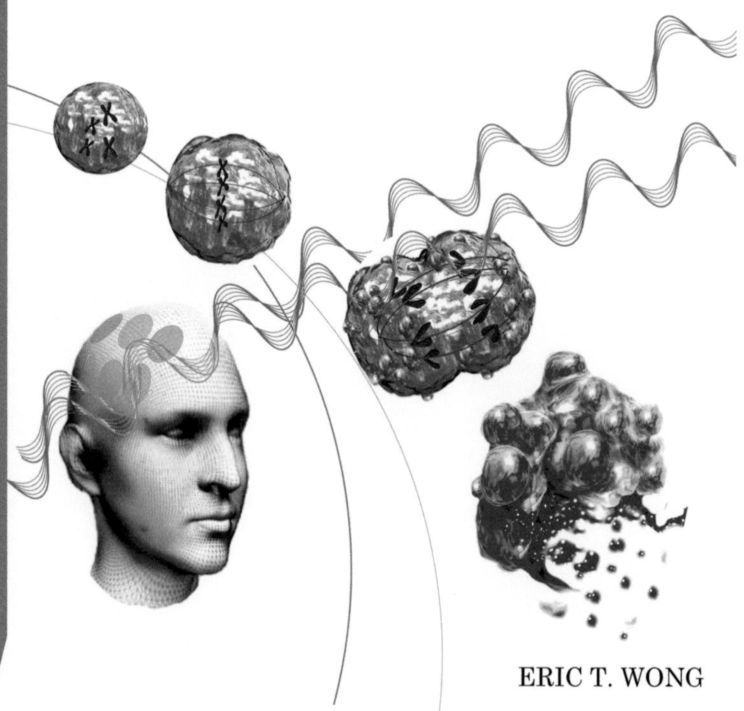

Eric T. Wong

Eric T. Wong
Editor

# Alternating Electric Fields Therapy in Oncology

## A Practical Guide to Clinical Applications of Tumor Treating Fields

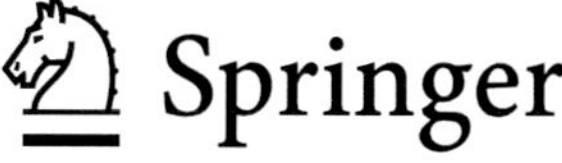

*Editor*
Eric T. Wong
Division of Neuro-Oncology
Department of Neurology
Beth Israel Deaconess Medical Center
Boston, MA, USA

ISBN 978-3-319-30574-5 ISBN 978-3-319-30576-9 (eBook)
DOI 10.1007/978-3-319-30576-9

Library of Congress Control Number: 2016953732



Printed on acid-free paper

This Springer imprint is published by Springer Nature
The registered company is Springer International Publishing AG Switzerland

# Preface

> "Questioning our own beliefs in this way (...challenging our assumptions...) isn't easy, but it is the first step in forming new, hopefully more accurate, beliefs."
>
> Duncan J. Watts in ***Everything is Obvious***

When Mike Ambrogi from Novocure sat down in my office for the first time in 2006 showing me a time-lapse video, I was mesmerized by the cells "blowing up" under the influence of alternating electric fields or Tumor Treating Fields. At that time, he was trying to enlist sites to participate in Novocure's EF-11 phase III clinical trial comparing a device that emits these fields to chemotherapy for recurrent glioblastoma. The device was strange because it required shaving of the patient's head and applying to the scalp four transducer arrays and each one had a set of nine ceramic disks. There were wires connecting the arrays to a box that generated the electric fields. At that time, *The Matrix* and its sequels were topping the box office and permeating popular culture. I was wondering whether or not this was the beginning of a brain-machine interface for the treatment of brain cancer. But in all seriousness, two killer questions came to my mind after seeing the video that led to our research team's long-term commitment in this scientific exploration: (1) Did the alternating electric fields at 200 kHz ($10^3$ Hz) permeate from the surface of the scalp into the brain, and (2) what was the biological mechanism causing the cells to blow up? The answer to the first question was easier to find. This took me back to my undergraduate senior design project at UPenn's engineering school when I was working on optimizing electronic circuits in the gigahertz ($10^9$ Hz) range or the microwave part of the electromagnetic spectrum. One thing I learned from the experience was that whether or not an alternating signal bounces from or penetrates into an object really depends on its frequency. Fortunately, a paper published in 1996 had a "spec sheet" on the dielectric properties of skull, gray matter, and white matter in the kilohertz range. It showed that the permittivity (the ability to hold charges) and conductivity (the ability to pass charges) of the three structures are similar and all of parameters are within an order of magnitude from each other, suggesting that the electric fields at 200 kHz can permeate skull, gray matter, and white matter as if they were one continuous medium. This is similar to light passing through a window into your living room—you are able to read a book either inside or outside of your home.

The second question was harder to address because there was still a lot of uncertainty in the cell biology effects from the electric fields at 200 kHz. I took the video on Tumor Treating Fields to Lew Cantley's lab in the Division of Signal Transduction and showed it to multiple postdoctoral researchers there. There were a lot of comments like "cool," "interesting," "far out" … etc. Ken Swanson was one of them but, like me, he was also mesmerized by the video. He reviewed the video multiple times over a few days, like a child watching cartoons over and over as if each time was a new experience. He made one very important observation and pointed out that after the cells underwent violent blebbing, they spread out and went back into the tissue culture—they did not die or dissociate from the dish. We both concluded that more cell biology experiments needed to be done and, after obtaining an unrestricted sponsored research agreement, we discovered that the blebbing process is a result of disrupted septins causing disorganized cytokinesis when cells transition from metaphase to anaphase. The aftermath of this disruption is aberrant mitotic exit, asymmetric chromosome segregation, and eventually immunogenic cell death. At about the same time, the results of the EF-11 trials came out and the device was approved by the U.S. Food and Drug Administration in 2011 for use in patients with recurrent glioblastoma and, later in 2015, for newly diagnosed glioblastoma.

Ed Lok is the third member of our research team, and he is the driving force behind our understanding of the electric field distributions in the brain. He has degrees in physics from college and radiation physics from graduate school, and he now works as a full-time medical physicist. He is intensely interested in the application of medical physics in medicine and after 8 years on our team he is still determined to figure out the most accurate method for delineating these tumor treating electric fields in the brain.

I learned an invaluable lesson while performing this translational research. I realized how different the training of a physician is from that of a research scientist, regardless of the subject of investigation such as addressing unanswered questions in basic biological sciences or testing the efficacy of new medical treatments. A clinician's job is to properly diagnose and appropriately treat a patient's ailment, and this is done by taking a careful history and observing the patient, as well as using whatever diagnostic tests that are available to arrive at a set of diagnoses that best fit the available data. Through a process of elimination, which is a weighted assessment based on the clinical acumen of that physician or the results from additional diagnostic tests, the clinician will then arrive at a "best fit" diagnosis and then treat the disease accordingly. In contrast, an investigator's job is find answers to an unexplained observation or question. It is dangerous to go into a scientific investigation with a preconceived notion of outcome. Quite often, these preconceived ideas reside in our subconscious and they can wholeheartedly interfere with the proper interpretation of observations and empirical data, particularly when conflicting results are present. In my experience, a seasoned scientist or investigator is more receptive to outlandish ideas than clinicians, probably because the latter are conditioned in a Pavlovian fashion to find the "best fit" explanation. Therefore, as commented in Duncan Watts' book, ***Everything is Obvious***, questioning my own beliefs is essential in forming new, and hopefully more accurate, beliefs.

Boston, MA, USA Eric T. Wong, MD

# Acknowledgements

This is the first textbook on alternating electric fields in oncology—also known as Tumor Treating Fields—and I certainly could not have accomplished this work without the help of others. I thank my longtime collaborators, Ken Swanson and Ed Lok, for working with me on this subject for nearly a decade, as well as Novocure for providing an unrestricted sponsored research agreement so that we can address some of the fundamental questions on Tumor Treating Fields in our laboratory. I am also indebted to contributors of this book who found the time and energy to write chapters that are essential for current understanding of this anti-cancer treatment. My neurology chief of service at Beth Israel Deaconess Medical Center Clif Saper is equally supportive of my clinical and research endeavors. Although protected time is often a sought after commodity in academic medicine, changes in the health care environment and federal funding structure in the United States make it increasingly challenging. But I am fortunate to have extraordinary support at work and at home. Deborha Cooper, Julianne Bloom, and Loretta Barron are the staff members in the brain tumor clinic who have been working with me for over a decade and they are instrumental in helping me care for a large number of complex patients. Lastly, my wife Ling and my daughter Erika are the two individuals at home who make my after-work moments enjoyable, not to mention my wife's green chiffon cake and her gourmet Trung Nguyên Vietnamese coffee that really improve my ability to do academic work. Likewise, I totally enjoy being a coach in Erika's Math League program in elementary school, where I have an opportunity to explain abstract concepts to her and her friends while simultaneously watching them learn.

There are a number of other individuals who helped me tremendously in compiling this book. Those who made this work possible include Greg Sutorius and Mariah Gumpert from Springer who helped with the publishing process, Janlyn Murphy who proofread a number of chapters, and Barbara Beiss from Novocure who helped me to get permission for a number of copyrighted figures from various publishers.

Kisa Zhang was instrumental in creating the beautiful digital artwork, and she was especially good at translating concepts in physics and biology into visual art. Finally, my patient Tom DesFosses, a brain tumor survivor, and his wife Judy DesFosses are two individuals who provided me unwavering support for nearly a decade with their optimism and their fundraising efforts in *A Reason to Ride* annual bikeathon.

# Contents

# Contributors

**Manmeet S. Ahluwalia, M.D.** Burkhardt Brain Tumor and Neuro-Oncology Center, Neurological Institute, Cleveland Clinic, Cleveland, OH, USA

**John DeNigris** Morsani College of Medicine, University of South Florida, Tampa, FL, USA

**Nidhi Gera, Ph.D.** Department of Biological Chemistry and Molecular Pharmacology, Harvard Medical School, Boston, MA, USA

**Andrew A. Kanner, M.D.** Stereotactic Radiosurgery Unit, Department of Neurosurgery, Tel Aviv Sourasky Medical Center, Tel Aviv University, Tel Aviv, Israel

**Mario E. Lacouture, M.D.** Oncodermatology Service, Memorial Sloan Kettering Cancer Center, New York, NY, USA

**Edwin Lok, M.S.** Division of Neuro-Oncology, Department of Neurology, Beth Israel Deaconess Medical Center, Boston, MA, USA

**Minesh P. Mehta, M.D.** Department of Radiation Oncology, University of Maryland Medical Center, Baltimore, MD, USA

**Pedro C. Miranda, Ph.D.** Institute of Biophysics and Biomedical Engineering, Faculdade de Ciências, Universidade de Lisboa, Lisboa, Portugal

**Maciej M. Mrugala, M.D., Ph.D., M.P.H.** Department of Neurological Surgery, University of Washington and Fred Hutchinson Cancer Research Center, Seattle, WA, USA

Department of Neurology, University of Washington and Fred Hutchinson Cancer Research Center, Seattle, WA, USA

Department of Medicine, University of Washington and Fred Hutchinson Cancer Research Center, Seattle, WA, USA

**Zvi Ram, M.D.** Department of Neurosurgery, Tel Aviv Sourasky Medical Center, Tel Aviv University, Tel Aviv, Israel

**Aaron M. Rulseh, M.D., Ph.D.** Department of Radiology, Na Homolce Hospital, Prague, Czech Republic

Department of Radiology, First Medical Faculty, Charles University in Prague, Prague, Czech Republic

**Jacob Ruzevick, M.D.** Department of Neurological Surgery, University of Washington and Fred Hutchinson Cancer Research Center, Seattle, WA, USA

**Erno Sajo, Ph.D.** Department of Physics, University of Massachusetts Lowell, Lowell, MA, USA

**Kenneth D. Swanson, Ph.D.** Division of Neuro-Oncology, Department of Neurology, Beth Israel Deaconess Medical Center, Boston, MA, USA

**Josef Vymazal, M.D., D.Sc.** Department of Radiology, Na Homolce Hospital, Prague, Czech Republic

Department of Neurology, First Medical Faculty, Charles University in Prague, Prague, Czech Republic

**Cornelia Wenger, Dr.techn.** Institute of Biophysics and Biomedical Engineering, Faculdade de Ciências, Universidade de Lisboa, Lisboa, Portugal

**Eric T. Wong, M.D.** Division of Neuro-Oncology, Department of Neurology, Beth Israel Deaconess Medical Center, Boston, MA, USA

Department of Physics, University of Massachusetts Lowell, Lowell, MA, USA

# Chapter 1
# Cell Biological Effects of Tumor Treating Fields

**Nidhi Gera and Kenneth D. Swanson**

## Application of Electric Fields to Patient Care

Electrotherapy involves the use of electrical energy for the treatment of medical conditions. Starting in the mid to late 1800s there was a fascination with the possible effects of electricity on the human body. This led to a proliferation of electricity-based devices that claimed to treat various maladies. While there were a limited number of cases where these devices led to the development of standard medical equipment, such as physiotherapeutic devices used to prevent muscle atrophy and cardiac defibrillators developed to stop arrhythmia, most early attempts proved to have little efficacy beyond possible placebo effects [1].

The biologic effects of electric fields within different tissues are dependent on both the intensity and frequency of the stimulating electric field or current. Different frequencies have vastly different biologic effects. For instance, at 1 kHz or lower, alternating electric fields cause depolarization of membrane potentials in excitable cells, such as neurons, cardiac myocytes, and muscle cells, via opening of voltage-gated ion channels [2–4]. Defibrillators, electro-shock therapy, and neuromuscular stimulation of muscles all rely on their ability of high intensity electric fields to induce membrane depolarization. In an early attempt to test whether electric fields were able to directly affect cellular physiology at a more molecular level, Rosenberg et al. [5] in 1965 at Michigan State University exposed *E. coli* cultures to electric fields generated by immersing platinum electrodes into the broth. This led to a

N. Gera, Ph.D.
Department of Biological Chemistry and Molecular Pharmacology,
Harvard Medical School, Boston, MA 02115, USA

K.D. Swanson, Ph.D. (✉)
Division of Neuro-Oncology, Department of Neurology,
Beth Israel Deaconess Medical Center, Boston, MA 02215, USA
e-mail: kswanson@bidmc.harvard.edu



E.T. Wong (ed.), *Alternating Electric Fields Therapy in Oncology*,
DOI 10.1007/978-3-319-30576-9_1

reduction in cell division, but not cell growth, resulting in the elongated growth of the bacteria [5]. This suggested that their cell division was sensitive to perturbation by electric fields. However, it was subsequently demonstrated that the media contained cisplatin produced *de novo* upon passing electric current through the platinum electrodes during the course of the experiment. This was found to be responsible for the observed growth effects [6]. Fortuitously, while this attempt failed to demonstrate the effects of electric fields on cellular function, it was later found that cisplatin, produced by the electrodes during this experiment, had potent anti-mitotic effects on cancer cells and is now a commonly used cancer chemotherapeutic [7].

## Tumor Treating Fields

Dr. Yorum Palti, emeritus professor at the Rappaport Institute in Israel, developed a technology to deliver electric fields to tumor cells without such chemical alterations to the media by using insulated electrodes. In these experiments, cell viability was profoundly affected at frequencies between 100 and 250 kHz. More precise measurements of cell viability revealed a reasonably tight peak of this cytotoxic effect in all cell types tested between 150 and 200 kHz, with little or no effect being detectable at frequencies below 50 kHz or above 500 kHz. The effect of these alternating electric fields also increased with field intensity. Given their cytotoxic effects these alternate electric fields within this frequency range were referred to as Tumor Treating Fields (TTFields) [8, 9]. Cells exposure to TTFields within mitosis exhibited violent membrane blebbing [9] and exposed cells have also been shown to be increased in volume [10]. While possible, no other clearly defined effects on cellular physiology have yet been reported for TTFields. When treated cell cultures were stained for tubulin and DNA it was found that spindle elements and the mitotic chromosomal order were disrupted. One of the more enigmatic features of TTFields' biophysical impact on cells is that the incident angle to the mitotic plate dictates the magnitude of cellular damage. When the TTFields were aligned perpendicular to the plane of division, cells were relatively unaffected, whereas cells exhibited a higher degree of mitotic failure if the TTFields were oriented parallel to the plane of division [9].

TTFields-induced mitotic disruption occurs coincident with cells exit from metaphase. Early reports showed that cells exposed to TTFields exhibited increased time in mitosis [9, 11]. Our laboratory showed that there was no gross perturbation in transit that would suggest a block during metaphase exit [12]. We found that the degradation of both cyclin B and securin [13], which occurs at the end of metaphase, was similar in both TTFields- and sham-treated cultures. Staining of microtubule in metaphase cells also appears grossly intact. Because normal exit from metaphase is triggered by the capture of microtubule ends within the metaphase spindle by kinetochores of chromatids that are properly aligned to metaphase plate (see below), our data suggest that metaphase spindle formation and function are unperturbed. However, there was a measurable increase in cells with 4N DNA content following TTFields treatment and persistence in phosphorylated Histone H3 levels, which is usually dephosphorylated in telophase [12, 13]. Further, time-lapse microscopy of cells stained with a vital DNA dye, allowing the accurate staging of mitosis, revealed that cells treated with TTFields undergo membrane blebbing at the time of metaphase exit [12]. Together, these data strongly suggest that TTFields-treated cells transit normally through metaphase but are disrupted in anaphase due to the violent mitotic blebbing and that leads to aberrant mitotic exit.

TTFields have also been shown to affect the growth of tumor in animal models and human cancers. Treating mice with a number of injected tumors grown from different cell lines including CT26 colon adenocarcinoma, B16/F1 melanoma, Lewis lung carcinoma, F-98 rat glioma, and the highly invasive VX2 carcinoma in rabbits were all shown to undergo tumor regression when TTFields were administered by electrodes placed outside of the body [8, 9, 14, 15]. Interestingly, when the VX2 tumors implanted under the kidney capsule were treated with TTFields delivered only to the abdomen, avoiding the lungs, there was also a marked decrease in lung metastasis compared to sham-treated animals. This suggests that TTFields may have affected either the metastatic potential of the tumor cells, or influenced host immune response against them [14]. These studies demonstrated that TTFields could penetrate the body and affect cellular physiology. This preclinical work led to TTFields testing against human gliomas and a successful phase III clinical trial [16].

Chen et al. [17] also applied similar intermediate frequency of alternating electric fields to B16/F10 melanoma cells both in culture and on tumors developed from flank injection in mice. Their data also showed the inhibition of cellular proliferation in culture and induction of apoptosis in an electrical intensity- and frequency-dependent manner similar to that reported above for TTFields. When they applied these fields to B16/F10 tumors grown in mice they significantly inhibited tumor growth, increased apoptosis by TUNEL staining, and increased mouse survival. Interestingly, they also found that CD34-positive cell numbers were reduced in the treated tumors, indicating an effect on the tumor microvasculature [17]. Beyond being necessary for perfusion of oxygen and nutrients into the tumor bed, tumor endothelium has been implicated in supporting the intratumoral immune inhibitory environment [18, 19]. This suggests that TTFields may target proliferating tumor endothelial cells, and the destruction of these cells may play a major role in contributing to tumor regression.

## Basis of Vulnerability to Tumor Treating Fields During Mitosis

Since TTFields affect cells during mitosis, this suggests a specific vulnerability to them may exist in this phase of the cell cycle. The cell cycle is a regimented process that controls cellular growth and proliferation. Biomass accumulation and cellular growth occur during interphase, which is subdivided into $G_1$, S, and $G_2$ phases. Non-mitotic and post-mitotic cells exist in a state referred to as $G_0$. Cell division and daughter cell production occur during mitosis, or M phase, which is further subdivided into prometaphase, metaphase, anaphase, and telophase. During the lengthy period of interphase, enzymatically-driven metabolic processes dominate cellular behavior with most structural requirements being involved in migration and cell polarization. However, during mitosis, which only lasts approximately 90 minutes in most cultured cells, the dominant cellular processes are almost completely dependent upon the rapid assemblage and function of mitosis-specific protein structures. Unlike the structures that cells depend on during interphase, these mitosis-specific structures require high levels of spatial and temporal precision for their functions. Therefore, while interphase is a highly anisotropic stage, M phase depends on a significant structural ordering at the molecular level in order to achieve successful cell division. This fact likely makes mitosis more susceptible to the electromotive disruption of TTFields than interphase (Fig. 1.1).

The accumulation of newly condensed chromosomes at the midline is dependent on rapid assembly of the highly ordered microtubule structures of the metaphase spindle produced early by the cell after it enters mitosis. During prometaphase, chromosomal material condenses into individually identifiable sister chromatid pairs. In order to migrate to the metaphase plate, the chromatids attach to the metaphase spindle microtubules and move towards the midline through the action of Kinesin motor proteins (Fig. 1.2A) [20]. Once there, the kinetochores within the centromeric regions of each sister chromatid captures microtubules end that are arrayed along the central plane of the dividing cell. This ensures that all chromatid pairs are aligned on the metaphase plate with their constituent kinetochores oriented towards the respective pole of each forming daughter cell. This is necessary to ensure the inheritance of a full complement of chromosomes in each daughter cell. The capture of the microtubules by the paired kinetochores creates physical tension between them that terminates the signals responsible for preventing premature metaphase exit [21]. Since a single pair of unattached kinetochores generates sufficient signal to prevent metaphase exit, the capture of the last kinetochore is required for mitotic progression from metaphase to anaphase. Final kinetochore capture triggers mitotic exit by permitting the rapid and irreversible activation of the anaphase promoting complex (APC/C) ubiquitin ligase activity (Fig. 1.2B). Active APC/C targets the $G_2$ Cyclin, Cyclin B, and Securin for destruction. Cyclin B is the allosteric activator of the Cyclin-dependent kinase 1 (CDK1) whose activity initiates mitosis and drives cells into metaphase while simultaneously inhibiting processes necessary for anaphase. Securin acts to inhibit the protease Seperase that cleaves the Cohesen protein complexes. This cleavage, along with CDK1 inactivation is necessary for the sister chromatids at the mitotic plate to separate and migrate towards the poles of their respective forming daughter cells [22]. Since APC/C is only activated following the capture of the last kinetochore, metaphase exit requires proper microtubule spindle formation and function [23].

Within anaphase, two additional highly ordered structures form, perform their precisely choreographed functions, and are then rapidly disassembled. The anaphase central spindle is a structure consisting of two parallel arrays of microtubules that are joined at the newly formed midline and extend away from each other. This structure is developed to perform two vital functions within minutes of entry into anaphase. During this time, the anaphase spindle pushes the newly formed chromosomes towards the poles of the forming daughter cells. At the same time, the mid-

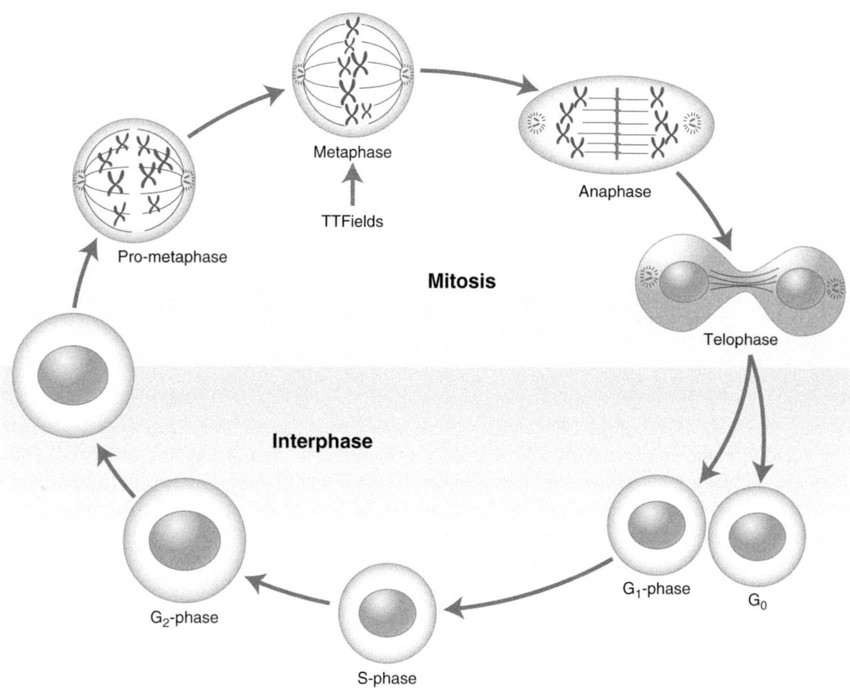


**Fig. 1.1** TTFields affect cells during the metaphase to anaphase transition. Dividing cells obtain biomass during interphase and form daughter cells during mitosis. Most of the processes that are essential to cells in interphase are metabolic in nature, many of which function to produce biomass in the form of protein, lipid, and DNA needed for division. On the other hand, mitosis involves the orderly mechanical segregation of daughter chromosomes and division of the parental cell cytoplasm in order to form two independent cells. Mitosis depends on a series of events driven through prometaphase, metaphase, anaphase, and telophase that must be executed with precision in order to ensure that each daughter cell inherits a full and equal complement of the parental genome after it has been duplicated during S phase. Cells that exit mitosis can remain in the cell cycle and enter the $G_1$ state or exit the cell cycle and enter the $G_0$ state. The actions of TTFields cause disruption of cells around the time of metaphase exit where the coordination of these mitotic processes is most critical.

line also plays an essential role in the organization and regulation of the third essential mitotic structure, the cytokinetic cleavage furrow (CCF) [24]. This structure contains powerful actinomycin motor elements that are arranged in a circumference around the equatorial cleavage plane of the dividing cells and is responsible for rapidly cinching the CCF closed during cytokinesis. Significantly, processes within anaphase must be initiated and completed within a short time frame (approximately 10 minutes), and coordinated with each other precisely. This strongly suggests a potential for vulnerability to the electromotive forces generated by TTFields exists during anaphase (Fig. 1.2C). There are a number of proteins within the anaphase spindle midline and the CCF that regulate their organization and contraction, including the centralspindalin complex, composed of KIF23 and MgcRacGAP, which are substrates for phosphorylation by polo-like kinase 1 (PLK1). This phos-

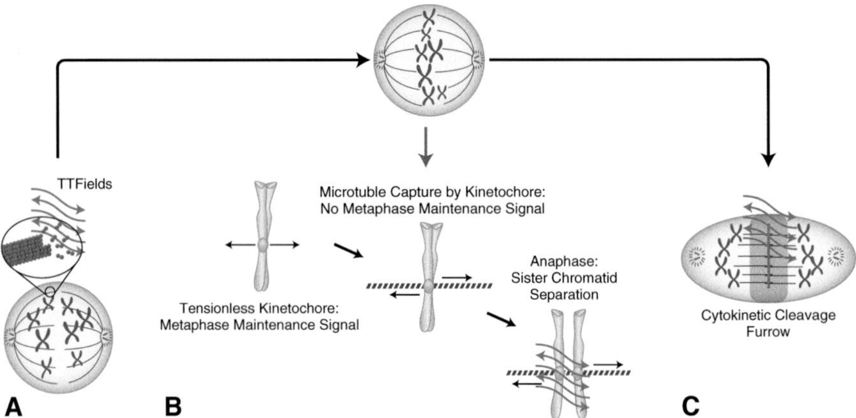


**Fig. 1.2** Different stages of mitosis represent different potential points of vulnerability to TTFields. TTFields may perturb mechanically critical processes that are specifically required during mitotic progression, such as the rapid polymerization and/or stability of microtubules in the metaphase spindle (**A**). The division of sister chromosomes subsequent to kinetochore capture of metaphase spindle microtubules requires the formation of the anaphase spindle, which may also be susceptible to perturbation by TTFields (**B**). The protein structures that underlay the cytokinetic furrow are also potential targets for TTFields disruption (**C**).

phorylation creates a binding site for the RhoGEF ECT2 resulting in its recruitment to the spindle midline [25]. ECT2 further binds to the adaptor protein Anillin which in turn binds to the heterotrimeric GTP binding protein Septin 2, 6, 7 complex [26]. ECT2-bound Anillin is required for the stability of the anaphase spindle midline, which becomes disordered upon its depletion [27]. ECT2 is subsequently delivered from the anaphase spindle midline to the CCF, where it is instrumental in directing the localization and regulation of its function during cytokinesis [28]. Upon its recruitment to the CCF, the Septin heterotrimers oligomerize into a highly ordered cytoskeleton-like scaffold that functions to recruit and organize the actinomyosin contractile elements required for furrow ingression and separation of the daughter cells [26, 27, 29–32]. In addition to its function within the CCF, Septins also crosslink F-actin bundles within the submembranous actin cytoskeleton [33–36]. This structure must possess adequate rigidity to withstand the hydrostatic pressures generated by ingression of the cytokinetic furrow. Failure to restrain these forces results in rupture of the connection between cytoskeleton and the overlying plasma membrane which leads to membrane blebbing [33].

## Molecular Targets of Tumor Treating Fields

There are several features that a molecular target of TTFields would need to possess in order to produce the observed cellular disruption during mitosis. First, alternating electric fields are likely to act by inducing movement of their molecular targets. This suggests that the presence of high molecular charges on proteins will act to align them

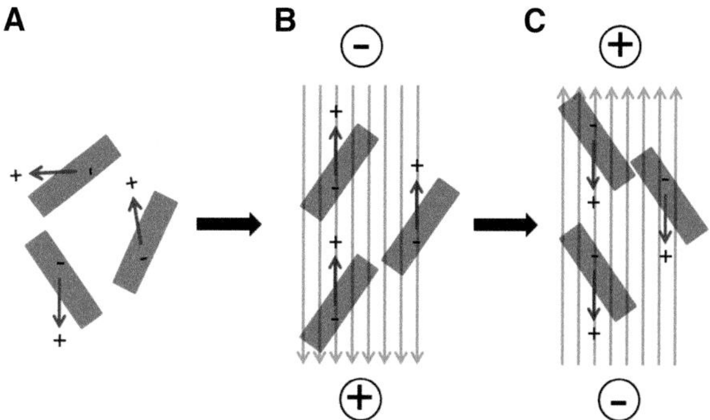


**Fig. 1.3** Protein dipole behavior in alternating electric fields. Some proteins possess dipole moments that form positive and negative poles within their structures due to differential densities of positive and negatively charged amino acid residues distributed on their surfaces (**A**). Within electric fields, the charges on the dipoles are oriented towards the opposite-charged field poles (**B**). As the poles of an alternating electric field are reversed, the orientation of the dipole containing protein will simultaneously be re-oriented due to the attractive forces imposed by the opposite charges (**C**).

and possibly induce movement. Proteins possess complex charge structures on their surfaces that arise from the charges of their surface amino acid side chains. The arrangement of acidic and basic residues on the protein surface potentially results in regional separations of surface charges imparting dipole moments onto some proteins, which can be similar to that observed in bar magnets (Fig. 1.3A). Proteins possessing such dipole moments will align within an electric field so that each pole of its dipole will orient towards the oppositely charged pole (Fig. 1.3B). Therefore, the repolarization of the alternating fields is expected to induce a re-orientation to realign the protein dipoles (Fig. 1.3C). Thus, an alternating field would be expected to result in the rotation or induce torsion on intracellular proteins possessing sufficiently high dipole moments, provided that the time constant of rotation or torsion is shorter than the time set for changes in external polarity [9]. Another property that TTFields targets might possess that would explain the ability of alternating electric fields to perturb cell behavior would be the participation of the target protein in the assembly of higher ordered structures. This would result in the electromotive forces exerted by TTFields disrupting cellular process that depends on the integrity of such structures.

Some of the proteins that are critical for the proper progression through mitosis have sufficiently high dipole moments to suggest that they may be affected by TTFields, including α/β-tubulin and the mitotic Septin 2, 6, 7 complex (Fig. 1.4). α/β-Tubulin form the building blocks of microtubules. Taxanes are commonly used chemotherapeutic agents that bind and stabilize microtubules and can cause mitotic catastrophe [37]. The α/β-tubulin heterodimer possesses a high predicted dipole moment of 1660 Debyes (D) (PDB 1JFF, [38, 39]). Therefore, it is possible that TTFields interfere with a critical mitotic function performed by microtubules such as interfering with α/β-tubulin function [8, 9], including the formation and regulation of the metaphase and anaphase spindles [40, 41], or the astral microtubules that are required for CCF regulation [42].

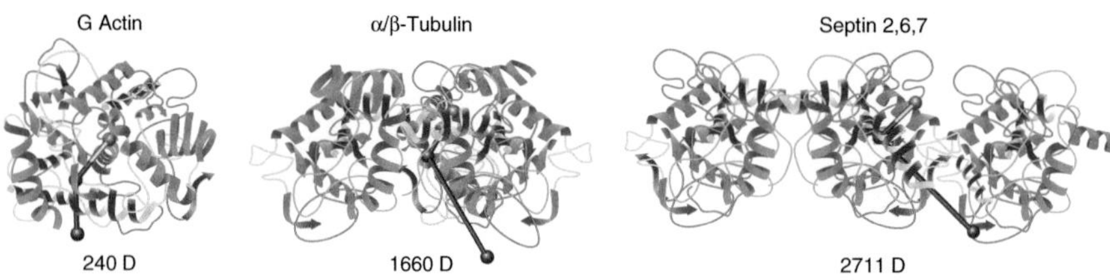


**Fig. 1.4** α/β-Tubulin and Septin 2, 6, 7 protein complexes possess high dipole moments. Crystal structures of G-actin, α/β-tubulin, and the Septin 2, 6, 7 complex with superimposed vectors representing the directionality and charge magnitude of their respective dipole moments. G-actin was chosen as a related protein example containing an insubstantial dipole moment.

Heterotrimeric Septin 2, 6, 7 also possesses a high predicted dipole moment of 2711 D (PDB 2QAG, [39, 43]). As described above, this Septin complex is required for functions that are necessary for the later stages of cell division. Septin 2, 6, 7 heterotrimers rapidly polymerize and structurally help to organize and coordinate the CCF activation during anaphase. Once recruited, they then oligomerize and organize the CCF above the equatorial cleavage plane by binding to F-actin filaments and spatially regulate myosin recruitment and activation. Depletion or mutation of ECT2 [44], Anillin [30] or Septin 7 [34] has been shown to result in defective cytokinesis and membrane blebbing. These studies strongly suggest that perturbation of any of the structural/regulatory elements during anaphase leads to aberrant mitotic exit similar to that observed in TTFields-treated cells. Septins also interact with both microtubules and several microtubule interacting proteins that influence microtubule positioning and stability during interphase and mitosis [45]. Therefore, perturbation of either Septin or α/β-tubulin may perturb the function of microtubules. Unlike the cases of cell cycle arrest induced by pharmacologic interventions, such as errors or damages that initiate the $G_1$/S, $G_2$/M, or spindle assembly check point (SAC), catastrophic errors that occur after the cell has committed to anaphase are unlikely to be correctable [46].

Supporting the hypotheses that TTFields induce mitotic catastrophe via a perturbation of Septin function, Septin localization to the anaphase spindle midline and cleavage furrow, as well as its reassociation with microtubules upon cell spreading, are significantly perturbed in cells exposed to TTFields [12]. The perturbation of the Septin complex being involved in the cellular response to TTFields is attractive due to its particularly high dipole moment and its known roles during mitosis, including the regulation of CCF function, actin bundle cross-linking, and organization of structures such as the cellular submembranous actin cytoskeleton that is required for its rigidity [33–36]. Further, depletion of Septin 7 by shRNA resulted in membrane blebbing during mitosis [9, 12, 34], as well as an increase in cell size [10, 34], similar to that seen with TTFields treatment. Therefore, this strongly suggests a mechanism of action where TTFields perturb mitosis by interfering with normal Septin localization and function during mitosis leading to membrane blebbing and aberrant mitotic exit. One of the structural features shared by both the $\alpha/\beta$-tubulin heterodimer and the Septin 2, 6, 7 heterotrimer is that the orientation of the dipole moment is predicted to be orthogonal to their longitudinal axis (Fig. 1.4), suggesting that as the polarity of the alternating field reverses, the effect on these proteins will be to induce "pinwheel-like" rotation around a central point within the respective proteins. It is therefore tempting to speculate that inducing such movement on the individual subunits may interfere significantly with their ability to coalesce into their respective higher ordered structures.

## Mitotic Effects of Tumor Treating Fields Result in Post-Mitotic Stress

The aberrant mitotic exit induced by TTFields resulted in a high degree of cellular stress, as indicated by increased cytoplasmic vacuoles, decrease in proliferation, and apoptosis [12]. Such aberrant mitotic exit has also been shown to lead to a p53-dependent $G_{0/1}$ cell cycle arrest. This is likely due to a failure to resolve the mitotic spindle apparatus, multiple centrioles, and/or the presence of supernumerary chromosomes [11, 47, 48]. p53-dependent $G_{0/1}$ arrest and apoptosis occurred more than 24 hours after TTFields exposure during mitosis [12]. This suggests the triggering of a p53-dependent mechanism by TTFields in response to mitotic catastrophe and aberrant mitotic exit. These data provide evidence that the efficacy of treatment may be influenced by tumor genetics.

## Potential for Immune Involvement in Tumor Treating Fields Mechanism of Action

TTFields may affect patient outcomes in different ways. As described above, TTFields are able to disrupt cells during mitosis and this phenomenon leads to aberrant mitotic exit and cell death. As in the case with spindle poisons, which trigger the spindle assembly checkpoints, cells affected by TTFields exhibit different fates including death in anaphase or aberrant exit from mitosis similar to mitotic slippage [49]. In this way, the mechanism of action may be similar to that proposed for other cancer therapies seeking to destroy tumor cells based on their inherent increased proliferation. This is thought to make them more susceptible to agents targeting dividing cells, such as spindle poisons.

Alternatively, there are several lines of evidence that support a possible immune dependency for TTFields efficacy. Senovilla et al. showed that tetraploid cells that are produced under experimental conditions that perturb mitotic exit exhibit the hallmarks of immunogenic cell death (ICD) [50]. This programmed form of cell death evokes an immune response against the dying cells through cell surface expression of the endoplasmic reticulum chaperone protein, Calreticulin, and the secretion of the cytokine/alarmins, HMGB1, and ATP [51, 52]. When injected into mice, these dying cells produced a protective immunization against subsequent challenge with the same tumor cell line [50]. Additionally, it has been recently demonstrated that cells made tetraploid by pharmacologic manipulation also express NKG2D and DNAM ligands on their surfaces that act to provoke their clearance by NK cells [53]. Cells that are exposed to TTFields have been shown to also exhibit cellular responses that are consistent with ICD including the cell surface expression of Calreticulin and secretion of HMGB1 [13]. Kirson et al. [14] showed that a brief 5-week TTFields treatment of subrenal capsule injected VX2 tumor in rabbits markedly reduced subsequent metastatic spread to the lungs. Examination of metastatic tumors in the lungs of these TTFields-treated rabbits showed a significant increase in immune infiltrates. This likely indicates a requirement for increased immune protective stroma for tumors that are capable of developing in these animals [14]. In the pivotal EF-11 trial that led to U.S. Food and Drug Administration approval for TTFields treatment of recurrent glioblastoma [16], response typically occurred 6.6–9.9 months following the onset of treatment at which point responders exhibited rapid tumor regression [54]. This pattern of delayed response is also consistent with an immune mechanism of tumor rejection. Finally, clinical data strongly suggest that the use of dexamethasone, a potent immunosuppressive agent, is correlated with patent outcome. Subjects receiving higher than 4.1 mg per day survived significantly shorter than those with lower doses and only subjects in the EF-11 trial who met these criteria responded to treatment [54, 55].

## Summary

TTFields likely function by exerting electromotive force on intracellular proteins that both possess sufficiently high dipole moments to be affected by them and are required for critical mitotic functions. Cells exposed to TTFields during mitosis exhibit catastrophic membrane blebbing around the time of metaphase exit resulting in failure within anaphase. TTFields are able to interfere with either structural integrity and/or function of critical proteins necessary for mitotic progression. Once cells become compromised in anaphase, they are unable to exit mitosis normally and slip out of mitosis in the absence of division. Such cells are deranged and nonviable and this can trigger an immune response against them (Fig. 1.5). More research is required to translate these basic science observations into improving the clinical efficacy of TTFields for cancer treatment.

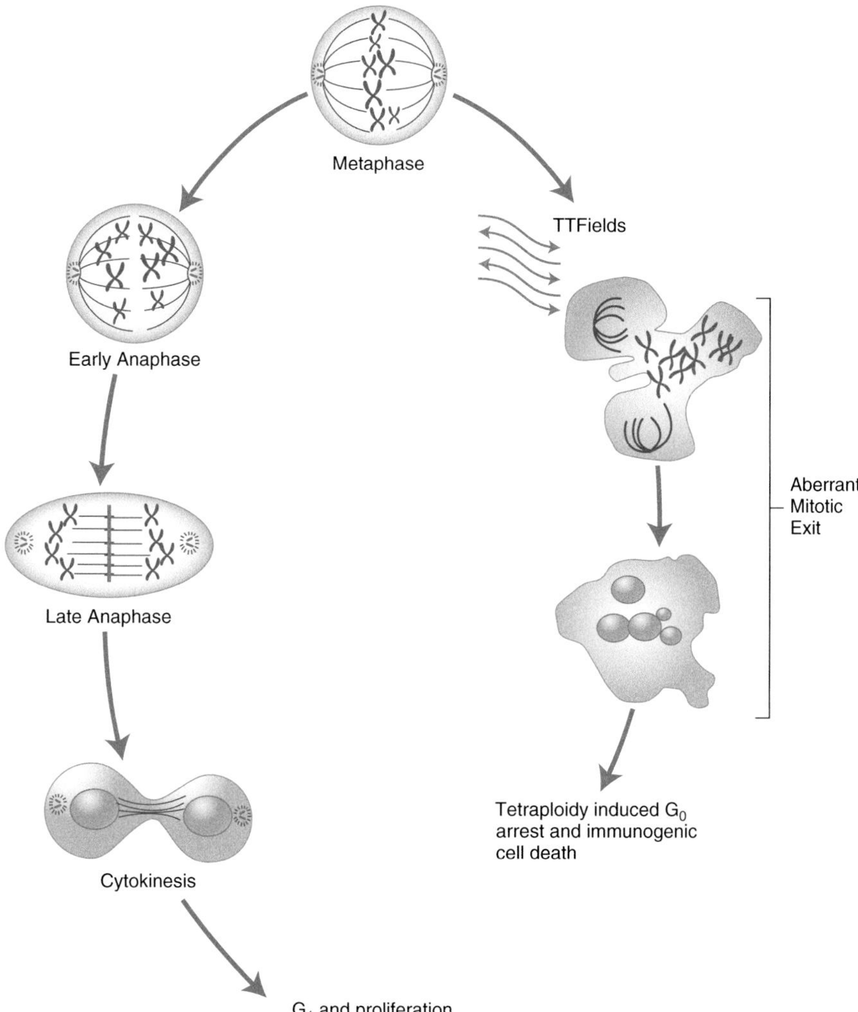


**Fig. 1.5** Model for cellular mechanism of action of TTFields. TTFields affect mitotic cells during anaphase resulting in membrane blebbing that perturbs cells during anaphase. This causes a failure of mitotic cleavage and aberrant exit from mitosis. Cells then enter $G_0$ arrest and progress to immunogenic cell death.

## References

1. Steinberg H. Electrotherapeutic disputes: the 'Frankfurt Council' of 1891. Brain. 2011;134(Pt 4):1229–43. Epub 2011/03/25.
2. Antoons G, Mubagwa K, Nevelsteen I, Sipido KR. Mechanisms underlying the frequency dependence of contraction and [Ca(2+)](i) transients in mouse ventricular myocytes. J Physiol. 2002;543(Pt 3):889–98. Epub 2002/09/17.

3. Posterino GS, Lamb GD, Stephenson DG. Twitch and tetanic force responses and longitudinal propagation of action potentials in skinned skeletal muscle fibres of the rat. J Physiol. 2000;527(Pt 1):131–7. Epub 2000/08/16.
4. Durand DM, Bikson M. Suppression and control of epileptiform activity by electrical stimulation: a review. Proc IEEE. 2001;89:1065–82.
5. Rosenberg B, Vancamp L, Krigas T. Inhibition of cell division in Escherichia coli by electrolysis products from a platinum electrode. Nature. 1965;205:698–9. Epub 1965/02/13.
6. Rosenberg B, Renshaw E, Vancamp L, Hartwick J, Drobnik J. Platinum-induced filamentous growth in Escherichia coli. J Bacteriol. 1967;93(2):716–21. Epub 1967/02/01.
7. Rosenberg B, VanCamp L, Trosko JE, Mansour VH. Platinum compounds: a new class of potent antitumour agents. Nature. 1969;222(5191):385–6. Epub 1969/04/26.
8. Kirson ED, Dbaly V, Tovarys F, Vymazal J, Soustiel JF, Itzhaki A, et al. Alternating electric fields arrest cell proliferation in animal tumor models and human brain tumors. Proc Natl Acad Sci U S A. 2007;104(24):10152–7. Epub 2007/06/07.
9. Kirson ED, Gurvich Z, Schneiderman R, Dekel E, Itzhaki A, Wasserman Y, et al. Disruption of cancer cell replication by alternating electric fields. Cancer Res. 2004;64(9):3288–95. Epub 2004/05/06.
10. Giladi M, Schneiderman RS, Porat Y, Munster M, Itzhaki A, Mordechovich D, et al. Mitotic disruption and reduced clonogenicity of pancreatic cancer cells in vitro and in vivo by tumor treating fields. Pancreatology. 2014;14(1):54–63. Epub 2014/02/22.
11. Giladi M, Schneiderman RS, Voloshin T, Porat Y, Munster M, Blat R, et al. Mitotic spindle disruption by alternating electric fields leads to improper chromosome segregation and mitotic catastrophe in cancer cells. Sci Rep. 2015;5:18046.
12. Gera N, Yang A, Holtzman TS, Lee SX, Wong ET, Swanson KD. Tumor treating fields perturb the localization of septins and cause aberrant mitotic exit. PLoS One. 2015;10(5):e0125269. Epub 2015/05/27.
13. Lee SX, Wong ET, Swanson KD. Disruption of cell division within anaphase by tumor treating electric fields (TTFields) leads to immunogenic cell death. Neuro-Oncol. 2013;15 Suppl 3:iii66–7.
14. Kirson ED, Giladi M, Gurvich Z, Itzhaki A, Mordechovich D, Schneiderman RS, et al. Alternating electric fields (TTFields) inhibit metastatic spread of solid tumors to the lungs. Clin Exp Metastasis. 2009;26(7):633–40. Epub 2009/04/24.
15. Kirson ED, Schneiderman RS, Dbaly V, Tovarys F, Vymazal J, Itzhaki A, et al. Chemotherapeutic treatment efficacy and sensitivity are increased by adjuvant alternating electric fields (TTFields). BMC Med Phys. 2009;9:1. Epub 2009/01/10.
16. Stupp R, Wong ET, Kanner AA, Steinberg D, Engelhard H, Heidecke V, et al. NovoTTF-100A versus physician's choice chemotherapy in recurrent glioblastoma: a randomised phase III trial of a novel treatment modality. Eur J Cancer. 2012;48(14):2192–202. Epub 2012/05/23.
17. Chen H, Liu R, Liu J, Tang J. Growth inhibition of malignant melanoma by intermediate frequency alternating electric fields, and the underlying mechanisms. J Int Med Res. 2012;40(1):85–94. Epub 2012/03/21.
18. Feng L, Sun X, Csizmadia E, Han L, Bian S, Murakami T, et al. Vascular CD39/ENTPD1 directly promotes tumor cell growth by scavenging extracellular adenosine triphosphate. Neoplasia. 2011;13(3):206–16. Epub 2011/03/11.
19. Lu J, Ye X, Fan F, Xia L, Bhattacharya R, Bellister S, et al. Endothelial cells promote the colorectal cancer stem cell phenotype through a soluble form of Jagged-1. Cancer Cell. 2013;23(2):171–85. Epub 2013/02/05.
20. Zhu C, Zhao J, Bibikova M, Leverson JD, Bossy-Wetzel E, Fan JB, et al. Functional analysis of human microtubule-based motor proteins, the kinesins and dyneins, in mitosis/cytokinesis using RNA interference. Mol Biol Cell. 2005;16(7):3187–99. Epub 2005/04/22.
21. Nezi L, Musacchio A. Sister chromatid tension and the spindle assembly checkpoint. Curr Opin Cell Biol. 2009;21(6):785–95. Epub 2009/10/23.
22. Oliveira RA, Hamilton RS, Pauli A, Davis I, Nasmyth K. Cohesin cleavage and Cdk inhibition trigger formation of daughter nuclei. Nat Cell Biol. 2010;12(2):185–92. Epub 2010/01/19.

23. Ge S, Skaar JR, Pagano M. APC/C- and Mad2-mediated degradation of Cdc20 during spindle checkpoint activation. Cell Cycle. 2009;8(1):167–71. Epub 2008/12/23.
24. D'Avino PP. How to scaffold the contractile ring for a safe cytokinesis—lessons from Anillin-related proteins. J Cell Sci. 2009;122(Pt 8):1071–9. Epub 2009/04/03.
25. Wolfe BA, Takaki T, Petronczki M, Glotzer M. Polo-like kinase 1 directs assembly of the HsCyk-4 RhoGAP/Ect2 RhoGEF complex to initiate cleavage furrow formation. PLoS Biol. 2009;7(5):e1000110. Epub 2009/05/27.
26. Field CM, Coughlin M, Doberstein S, Marty T, Sullivan W. Characterization of anillin mutants reveals essential roles in septin localization and plasma membrane integrity. Development. 2005;132(12):2849–60. Epub 2005/06/03.
27. Frenette P, Haines E, Loloyan M, Kinal M, Pakarian P, Piekny A. An anillin-Ect2 complex stabilizes central spindle microtubules at the cortex during cytokinesis. PLoS One. 2012;7(4):e34888. Epub 2012/04/20.
28. Gregory SL, Ebrahimi S, Milverton J, Jones WM, Bejsovec A, Saint R. Cell division requires a direct link between microtubule-bound RacGAP and Anillin in the contractile ring. Curr Biol. 2008;18(1):25–9. Epub 2007/12/26.
29. Straight AF, Field CM, Mitchison TJ. Anillin binds nonmuscle myosin II and regulates the contractile ring. Mol Biol Cell. 2005;16(1):193–201. Epub 2004/10/22.
30. Piekny AJ, Glotzer M. Anillin is a scaffold protein that links RhoA, actin, and myosin during cytokinesis. Curr Biol. 2008;18(1):30–6. Epub 2007/12/26.
31. Giansanti MG, Bonaccorsi S, Gatti M. The role of anillin in meiotic cytokinesis of Drosophila males. J Cell Sci. 1999;112(Pt 14):2323–34. Epub 1999/06/25.
32. Goldbach P, Wong R, Beise N, Sarpal R, Trimble WS, Brill JA. Stabilization of the actomyosin ring enables spermatocyte cytokinesis in Drosophila. Mol Biol Cell. 2010;21(9):1482–93. Epub 2010/03/20.
33. Gilden J, Krummel MF. Control of cortical rigidity by the cytoskeleton: emerging roles for septins. Cytoskeleton (Hoboken). 2010;67(8):477–86. Epub 2010/06/12.
34. Gilden JK, Peck S, Chen YC, Krummel MF. The septin cytoskeleton facilitates membrane retraction during motility and blebbing. J Cell Biol. 2012;196(1):103–14. Epub 2012/01/11.
35. Tooley AJ, Gilden J, Jacobelli J, Beemiller P, Trimble WS, Kinoshita M, et al. Amoeboid T lymphocytes require the septin cytoskeleton for cortical integrity and persistent motility. Nat Cell Biol. 2009;11(1):17–26. Epub 2008/12/02.
36. Hagiwara A, Tanaka Y, Hikawa R, Morone N, Kusumi A, Kimura H, et al. Submembranous septins as relatively stable components of actin-based membrane skeleton. Cytoskeleton (Hoboken). 2011;68(9):512–25. Epub 2011/07/30.
37. Sudakin V, Yen TJ. Targeting mitosis for anti-cancer therapy. BioDrugs. 2007;21(4):225–33. Epub 2007/07/14.
38. Lowe J, Li H, Downing KH, Nogales E. Refined structure of alpha beta-tubulin at 3.5 A resolution. J Mol Biol. 2001;313(5):1045–57. Epub 2001/11/09.
39. Felder CE, Prilusky J, Silman I, Sussman JL. A server and database for dipole moments of proteins. Nucleic Acids Res. 2007;35(Web Server issue):W512–21. Epub 2007/05/29.
40. Albertson R, Cao J, Hsieh TS, Sullivan W. Vesicles and actin are targeted to the cleavage furrow via furrow microtubules and the central spindle. J Cell Biol. 2008;181(5):777–90. Epub 2008/05/28.
41. D'Avino PP, Savoian MS, Glover DM. Cleavage furrow formation and ingression during animal cytokinesis: a microtubule legacy. J Cell Sci. 2005;118(Pt 8):1549–58. Epub 2005/04/07.
42. Rankin KE, Wordeman L. Long astral microtubules uncouple mitotic spindles from the cytokinetic furrow. J Cell Biol. 2010;190(1):35–43. Epub 2010/07/07.
43. Sirajuddin M, Farkasovsky M, Hauer F, Kuhlmann D, Macara IG, Weyand M, et al. Structural insight into filament formation by mammalian septins. Nature. 2007;449(7160):311–5. Epub 2007/07/20.
44. Su KC, Takaki T, Petronczki M. Targeting of the RhoGEF Ect2 to the equatorial membrane controls cleavage furrow formation during cytokinesis. Dev Cell. 2011;21(6):1104–15. Epub 2011/12/17.

45. Bowen JR, Hwang D, Bai X, Roy D, Spiliotis ET. Septin GTPases spatially guide microtubule organization and plus end dynamics in polarizing epithelia. J Cell Biol. 2011;194(2): 187–97. Epub 2011/07/27.
46. Huang HC, Shi J, Orth JD, Mitchison TJ. Evidence that mitotic exit is a better cancer therapeutic target than spindle assembly. Cancer Cell. 2009;16(4):347–58. Epub 2009/10/06.
47. Margolis RL, Lohez OD, Andreassen PR. G1 tetraploidy checkpoint and the suppression of tumorigenesis. J Cell Biochem. 2003;88(4):673–83. Epub 2003/02/11.
48. Ganem NJ, Pellman D. Limiting the proliferation of polyploid cells. Cell. 2007;131(3): 437–40. Epub 2007/11/06.
49. Orth JD, Loewer A, Lahav G, Mitchison TJ. Prolonged mitotic arrest triggers partial activation of apoptosis, resulting in DNA damage and p53 induction. Mol Biol Cell. 2012;23(4): 567–76. Epub 2011/12/16.
50. Senovilla L, Vitale I, Martins I, Tailler M, Pailleret C, Michaud M, et al. An immunosurveillance mechanism controls cancer cell ploidy. Science. 2012;337(6102):1678–84. Epub 2012/09/29.
51. Kepp O, Senovilla L, Vitale I, Vacchelli E, Adjemian S, Agostinis P, et al. Consensus guidelines for the detection of immunogenic cell death. Oncoimmunology. 2014;3(9):e955691. Epub 2015/05/06.
52. Kepp O, Tesniere A, Schlemmer F, Michaud M, Senovilla L, Zitvogel L, et al. Immunogenic cell death modalities and their impact on cancer treatment. Apoptosis. 2009;14(4):364–75. Epub 2009/01/16.
53. Acebes-Huerta A, Lorenzo-Herrero S, Folgueras AR, Huergo-Zapico L, Lopez-Larrea C, Lopez-Soto A, et al. Drug-induced hyperploidy stimulates an anti-tumor NK cell response mediated by NKG2D and DNAM-1 receptors. Oncoimmunology. 2015;5(2), e1074378.
54. Wong ET, Lok E, Swanson KD, Gautam S, Engelhard HH, Lieberman F, et al. Response assessment of NovoTTF-100A versus best physician's choice chemotherapy in recurrent glioblastoma. Cancer Med. 2014;3(3):592–602. Epub 2014/02/28.
55. Wong ET, Lok E, Gautam S, Swanson KD. Dexamethasone exerts profound immunologic interference on treatment efficacy for recurrent glioblastoma. Br J Cancer. 2015;113(2): 232–41. Epub 2015/07/01.

# Chapter 2
# Fundamental Physics of Tumor Treating Fields

**Edwin Lok and Erno Sajo**

Glioblastoma is one of the deadliest forms of brain tumor in humans, yielding a devastating and short survival of only 1 to 2 years [1]. Numerous treatment modalities have been made available to patients over the years to treat this terrible disease, often with only marginal prolongation of survival with a concomitant reduction of quality of life over the course of treatment and in many cases until death. In recent years, collaborative efforts at numerous institutions have been undertaken to investigate a novel noninvasive treatment using alternating electric fields, also known as Tumor Treating Fields (TTFields), and through randomized clinical trials this therapy has been shown to offer a survival advantage in patients with glioblastoma [2–4]. In some of the patients, TTFields were able to reduce tumor size and produce a radiologically visible response [5, 6]. Unlike conventional ionizing radiation, TTFields generated by the Optune® device do not induce direct damage to biomolecules, such as the DNA of the tumor as well as DNA of normal tissues [5, 6]. Also, in contrast to chemotherapy, the device generates electric fields targeting tumor regions, and enables the patient's own immune system to destroy actively dividing glioblastoma cells [7–9].

In order to better understand the clinical and biological effects of TTFields, this chapter is devoted to addressing the fundamental physics that governs these electric fields as generated by the Optune® device. Although a background in physics and mathematics is not required, having such will benefit the readers of this chapter and help them gain an appreciation for the data presented in subsequent chapters.

E. Lok, M.S. (✉)
Division of Neuro-Oncology, Department of Neurology,
Beth Israel Deaconess Medical Center, Boston, MA 02215, USA
e-mail: elok@bidmc.harvard.edu

E. Sajo, Ph.D.
Department of Physics, University of Massachusetts Lowell, Lowell, MA 01854, USA



E.T. Wong (ed.), *Alternating Electric Fields Therapy in Oncology*,
DOI 10.1007/978-3-319-30576-9_2

## The Fundamental Physics of Tumor Treating Fields

The biophysical effects of TTFields are governed by the fundamental laws of electricity and magnetism, namely Coulomb's law, Gauss's law, Ohm's law, and the continuity equation. The dynamic formulations of these laws (also known as electrodynamics) are different from the static versions (as in electrostatics) and they are important to our understanding of how TTFields, which are alternating electric fields at 150 to 200 kHz, induce mitotic disruption in cancer cells and antitumor effects in patients. While the Optune® device generates TTFields by two pairs of orthogonally positioned transducer arrays placed onto the surface of the patient's scalp, the degree of penetration and distribution of these fields from the scalp surface, passing through the calvarium, and into the brain depend on the local tissue properties including their electric conductivity (the ability to pass charges) and relative permittivity (the ability to hold charges) [9]. This is based on Gauss' law, Ohm's law, and the continuity equation that govern the electric field distribution in the human head. First, Coulomb's law describes the electric field strength at a test point located at a distance from a charge located in space and time (Fig. 2.1). Specifically, the field strength decreases in an inverse proportion to the square of the distance or $\frac{1}{r^2}$ from the charge, where $r$ is the radial distance between the test point and the charge.

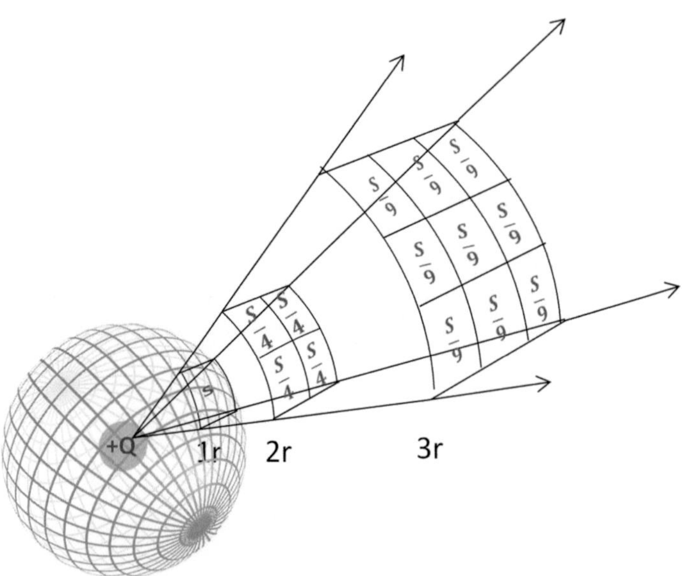


**Fig. 2.1** Coulomb's law expresses that the electric field strength drops off with the square of the distance between the charge and at a test point in space.

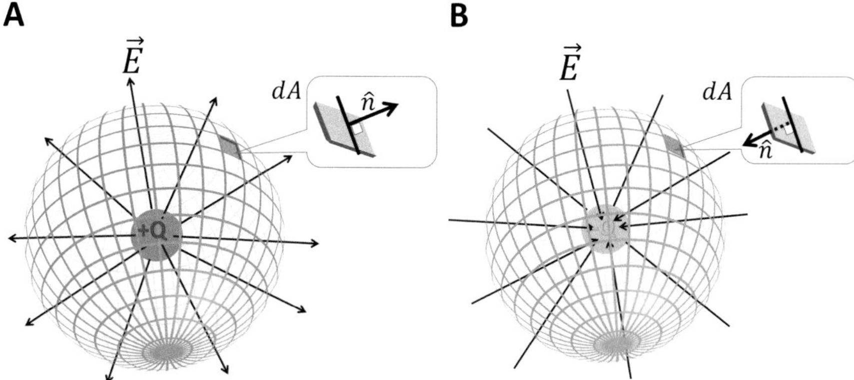


**Fig. 2.2** Gauss' law states that the electric flux $\Phi_E$ or the flow of electric field is equal to the net sum of the varying electric field $\vec{E}$ over a closed surface area in a volume that encloses all the charges, $Q$. Here, $\hat{n}$ represents the surface normal through a surface element $dA$. (**A**) The electric field lines generated by a positive point charge emanate from the center of the charge and impinge upon a Gaussian surface in an outward direction by convention. (**B**) The direction of electric field lines of a negative point charge point inward towards the center of charge by convention.

Gauss' law (Eq. 2.1a or Eq. 2.1b) can be derived from Coulomb's law, and it gives the relation between the electric charge and the electric field:

$$\nabla \cdot \vec{E} = \frac{\rho}{\varepsilon} \tag{2.1a}$$

$$\Phi_E = \oint \left(\vec{E} \cdot \hat{n}\right) dA = \frac{Q_{enclosed}}{\varepsilon_0} \tag{2.1b}$$

Gauss' law mathematically states that the divergence of the electric field, $\vec{E}$, is proportional to the space charge density $\rho$ and inversely proportional to the permittivity of tissue or media $\varepsilon$, which is traversed by the electric charge. Correspondingly, the divergence of $\vec{E}$ is the magnitude of electric field that passes through a cross-sectional area. When Gauss' law is written in its integral form (Eq. 2.1b), it states that the electric flux $\Phi_E$ or the flow of electric field is equal to the net sum of the varying electric field $\vec{E}$, over a closed surface area in a volume that encloses all the charges, $Q$ (Fig. 2.2). Here, $\hat{n}$ represents the surface normal through a surface element $dA$. Consequently, since the electric field is dependent upon the quantity of charge $Q$, it is also equal to the total charge enclosed divided by the permittivity of free space $\varepsilon_0$. Therefore, the magnitude of TTFields that traverses through various tissues in the brain, including the tumor, will change depending on the charge density and dielectric properties of the tumor and surrounding tissues.

Ohm's law (Eq. 2.2) is just as important as Gauss' law in determining the penetration and distribution of TTFields due to differences in the electrical properties of intracranial tissues. Ohm's law establishes that the electric current ($I$) is inversely proportional and dependent on the tissue's electric resistance ($R$) at a particular electric potential or voltage ($V$). The differences in resistance will vary according to the magnitude of the dielectric property of the tissue that the electric field traverses. It is possible to generalize Eq. 2.2 by replacing (1) the current, $I$, with the current density, $\vec{J}$; (2) the inverse of the electric resistance, $R$, with the tissue-dependent conductivity, $\sigma$; and (3) the electric potential with the electric field $\vec{E}$ (Eq. 2.4). This is made possible by satisfying Poisson's equation for electrostatics (Eq. 2.3), which states that the electric field is equivalent to the negative spatial gradient of the electric potential field $\varphi$. Hence, the greater the change in electric potential results in a more intense electric field. Since the change in electric potential on the surface of the scalp is significantly higher than that in intracranial tissue, scalp tissue therefore encounters a stronger electric field:

$$I = \frac{V}{R} \tag{2.2}$$

$$\vec{E} = -\nabla\varphi \tag{2.3}$$

$$\vec{J} = \sigma\vec{E} \tag{2.4}$$

Finally, the continuity equation describes the conservation of charges within a defined volume, where the divergence of electric current density $\vec{J}$ that passes through a cross-sectional area is equal to the loss of charge density from the volume over time (Eq. 2.5a). Loss of charge here may be interpreted as the negative rate of change in charge density over time, while a gain of charge is interpreted as the positive rate of change in charge density over time. This establishes the basis for charge conservation where charge is neither created nor destroyed. The continuity equation is a critical consideration for the computer modeling of electric field distribution within the brain, and this type of simulation provides the treating clinician a visualization of TTFields distribution in relation to the position of the glioblastoma [10]. Therefore, in this process, specifying the boundary conditions where charges are neither destroyed nor created is an important prerequisite:

$$\nabla\cdot\vec{J} = -\frac{\partial\rho}{\partial t} \tag{2.5a}$$

$$\nabla\cdot\left(-\sigma\nabla\varphi\right) = -\frac{\partial\rho}{\partial t} \tag{2.5b}$$

Utilizing Eqs. (2.3) and (2.4) the current density may be replaced by $-\sigma\nabla\varphi$, yielding Eq. 2.5b. Further, for alternating fields the tissue conductivity is related to the frequency-dependent permittivity, $\varepsilon(\omega)$, which will be discussed later in the chapter. The right-hand side of Eq. 2.5 may be set equal to 0 if it is assumed that the induction of electric currents by magnetic fields is negligible. This is known as the quasi-static approximation, which may be valid under the assumption that the wavelength of the applied field is much larger than the dimension of the object it traverses, i.e., the human brain [11–17]. In this way, many research groups using 10 kHz have assumed that $\partial\rho/\partial t = 0$ over a finite time step. Based on the dimensional argument, it appears that this approximation should be still valid at 200 kHz. However, a more rigorous solution that accounts for capacitive tissue effects and the brain's innate electric fields is to use the full Maxwell equations to solve for the electric field.

## Special Considerations for Time-Varying Properties of Tumor Treating Fields

Direct current implies an electric potential across a closed circuit that is constant over time, while alternating current implies a varying potential over an interval of time once the circuit is closed. For the purpose of describing the physical mechanism of TTFields action, we will only describe the applied electric potential by a standard sine wave as a function of time with no phase shift, where Ø = 0 (Eq. 2.6 and Fig. 2.3):

$$V(t) = V_{pk}\sin(2\pi ft + \phi) \tag{2.6}$$

$V_{pk}$ is the peak amplitude or peak voltage, $f$ is the frequency, and $\phi$ is the degree of phase shift. In order to compare the relative strength of different sinusoidal waves with different peak voltages, frequencies, and other parameters, the root mean

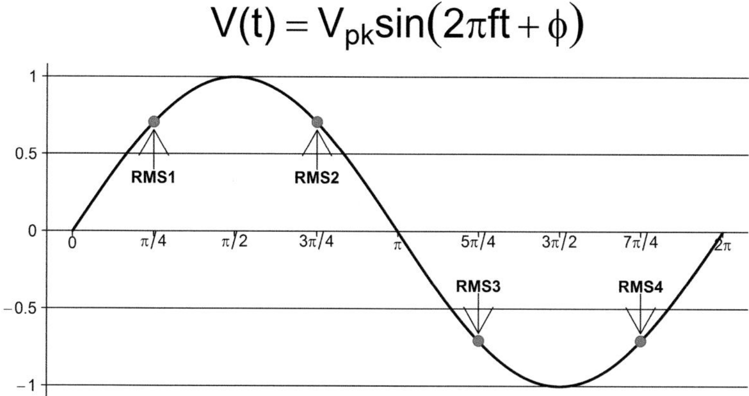


**Fig. 2.3** In order to compare the relative strength of different sinusoidal waves with different peak voltages, frequencies, and other parameters, the root mean square (RMS) value is most relevant because this is regarded as the average value of waveforms with alternating characteristics. For the sinusoidal voltage function $V(t) = V_{pk}\sin(2\pi ft + \phi)$, where $V_{pk}$ is the peak amplitude or peak voltage, $f$ is the frequency, and $\phi$ is the degree of phase shift, there are four RMS values, denoted as $V_{RMS1}$, $V_{RMS2}$, $V_{RMS3}$, and $V_{RMS4}$.

square (RMS) value is most relevant because this is regarded as the average value of waveforms with alternating characteristics. The RMS value is defined as the value of the amplitude divided by $\sqrt{2}$ . For the Optune® device, the electric fields that are generated consist of a continuous sinusoidal wave and, therefore, the RMS and peak-to-peak electric potentials are the most important voltage values on the curve.

The Optune® device by design produces a peak amplitude of roughly 50 V, operates at a frequency of 200 kHz, and has no phase shift. By definition, this sinusoidal function has four specific time points in one complete cycle during which the absolute value of the electric potential is at the RMS or average value. Because the definition of the RMS value for a sine wave is the amplitude divided by $\sqrt{2}$ , the four time points for the RMS value can be derived by specifying Eq. 2.6 with a peak voltage of 50 V to solve for $t$:

$$\frac{50}{\sqrt{2}}(V) = 50(V) \cdot \sin\left(2 \cdot \pi \cdot f(Hz) \cdot t(s) + 0\right) \quad \textit{Step } 1.$$

$$t_{RMS} = \frac{\sin^{-1}\left(\frac{1}{\sqrt{2}}\right)}{2\pi f} \quad \textit{Step } 2.$$

The term $\frac{\sin^{-1}\left(\frac{1}{\sqrt{2}}\right)}{2\pi}$ yields exactly $\frac{1}{8}$, indicating that the RMS value of the electric potential occurs at every $\frac{a_n}{8f}$ for $a_n = 2n - 1$ with $n = 1, 2, 3, 4$ per cycle. By inspection, the peak electric potential is irrelevant when solving for $t_{RMS}$ simply because it was cancelled out before reaching step 2. This clearly shows that $t_{RMS}$ is a characteristic of the frequency of the sine wave. This method is considered a simple and effective way for acquiring the four $t_{RMS}$ time points in any one cycle of the applied sine wave. These four $t_{RMS}$ time points are critically important for the visualization of the electric field distribution in the brain by computer modeling. The set of values below corresponds to the four generalized time points used to compute $V_{RMS}$ for a frequency of 200 kHz and a peak voltage of 50 V:

$$V_{RMS1} = 50(V) \cdot \sin\left(2 \cdot \pi \cdot f(Hz) \cdot \left(\frac{1}{8 \cdot 200{,}000}\right)(s) + 0\right) \cong 35.356V$$

$$V_{RMS2} = 50(V) \cdot \sin\left(2 \cdot \pi \cdot f(Hz) \cdot \left(\frac{3}{8 \cdot 200{,}000}\right)(s) + 0\right) \cong 35.356\ V$$

$$V_{RMS3} = 50(V) \cdot \sin\left(2 \cdot \pi \cdot f(Hz) \cdot \left(\frac{5}{8 \cdot 200{,}000}\right)(s) + 0\right) \cong -35.356\ V$$

$$V_{RMS4} = 50(V) \cdot \sin\left(2 \cdot \pi \cdot f(Hz) \cdot \left(\frac{7}{8 \cdot 200{,}000}\right)(s) + 0\right) \cong -35.356\ V$$

## Capacitive Response of Biological Tissues to Tumor Treating Fields

An accurate analysis of biological tissue response to the applied TTFields requires an understanding of the physical characteristics of a capacitor, which consists of a medium (also known as a dielectric) that retains charge over time. The dielectric medium may be any insulator material placed between conductive interfaces where charge is stored. Often, conductive media are associated with metals or metallic materials while insulators are likened to nonmetals, such as glass or air. However, when we rigorously analyze their properties, in practice they are neither perfect conductors nor perfect insulators. A perfect insulator essentially has the property where no electric charge or current may traverse through the material and thus its conductivity is equal to zero. By Eq. 2.4, the current density in this medium is 0 and therefore the electric field is 0 as well. Of course, in the real world any material considered an insulator has a finite threshold for dielectric breakdown, which occurs when a sufficiently high electric potential is applied across the medium at which it can no longer prevent charge transport. A classic example of this phenomenon would be lightning strike through air. When the electric field between the surface of the Earth and clouds in the atmosphere is large enough, the air's property as an insulator between the two interfaces temporarily breaks down due to a partial and propagating ionization of the gas from very high electric stress and thus a visible lightning strike is seen. The partial ionization of the gas can be explained further by considering that the potential energy applied across the gas exceeds the maximum threshold of the insulating capacity, which is defined by the dielectric strength of the gas medium. When saturated with charge, the insulator will momentarily act as a conductor, releasing a surge of energy where the charges flow to the ground at a near instant.

As the Optune® device applies a voltage across the head with a peak voltage of 50 V, there will be variations in the electric field distribution intracranially due to difference in material composition within different structures that are neither a perfect insulator nor a perfect conductor. Two important dielectric properties to consider are the electric conductivity ($\sigma$) and relative permittivity ($\varepsilon$). In general, the electric conductivity is derived from the electrical resistivity, and it governs the magnitude of the current density $\vec{J}$ for a uniformly applied electric field as previously described in Eq. 2.4. Specifically, the electric conductivity is the inverse of the electric resistivity. In the case of time-varying or alternating electric fields, the relative permittivity is a complex parameter (with real and imaginary parts); it is a function of the angular frequency and is referenced to the permittivity of vacuum or that of free space $\varepsilon_0$ as seen in Eq. 2.1b. Equation 2.7a shows the relative permittivity as a function of the alternating field's angular frequency ($\omega$) written in both the real and imaginary parts, where $i = \sqrt{-1}$ and $\omega = 2\pi f$ . A more realistic way of expressing Eq. 2.7a is one that forms a relationship between the relative permittivity and conductivity for linear isotropic materials, as Eq. 2.7b does:

$$\varepsilon_r(\omega) = \varepsilon_r^{'}(\omega) + i\varepsilon_r^{''}(\omega) \tag{2.7a}$$

$$\varepsilon_r(\omega) = \varepsilon_r^{'}(\omega) + i\frac{\sigma}{\omega\varepsilon_0} \tag{2.7b}$$

Unfortunately, biological tissues invariably exhibit nonlinear anisotropic behaviors, where Eqs. 2.7a and 2.7b must be modified and thus the relative permittivity stems from a generalized dielectric relaxation model as given by the Cole-Cole equation, Eq. 2.8 [18–20]:

$$\varepsilon_r(\omega) = \varepsilon_\infty + \frac{\varepsilon_s - \varepsilon_\infty}{1 + (i\omega\tau)^{1-\alpha}} \tag{2.8}$$

Here, $\varepsilon_\infty$ and $\varepsilon_s$ are the infinite-frequency and static permittivities, respectively, and $\tau$ is a time constant. $\alpha$ is the spectral shape parameter with values between 0 and 1 (Debye model). Real-world materials, including biological tissue, are dielectrics that to some extent have bound charges forming neutral atoms. When an electric field is applied, the material will become polarized proportional to the polarization density $\vec{P}$. These bound charges distort the electric field in the medium due to a retarding effect that is dependent on the dipole moments and the electric susceptibility of materials $\chi_e$, which describes the ability of a dielectric to be polarized (Fig. 2.4). It should be noted, however, that for anisotropic medium, $\chi_e$ is a tensor, a quantity written in a matrix form that expresses both its magnitude and direction. For linear homogeneous isotropic dielectrics, the polarization density is related to the electric field and it can be written as a function of time, as in Eq. 2.9a, or as a function of frequency, as in Eq. 2.9b:

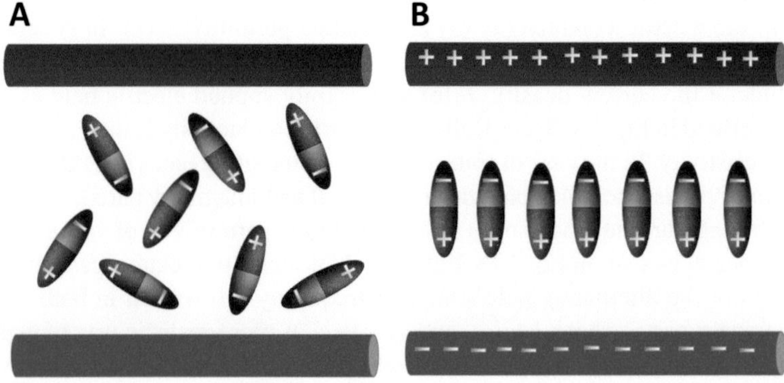


**Fig. 2.4** When an electric field is applied, the dipoles in (**A**) will become polarized proportional to the polarization density and align in a parallel fashion as in (**B**) to the applied electric field.

$$\vec{P}(t) = \varepsilon_0 \int_{-\infty}^{t} \chi_e(t-t')\vec{E}(t')dt' \tag{2.9a}$$

$$\vec{P}(\omega) = \varepsilon_0\, \chi_e(\omega)\vec{E}(\omega) \tag{2.9b}$$

Finally, the electric displacement field $\vec{D}$, which relates to the polarization density and the electric field, may be written in the frequency domain as in Eq. 2.10:

$$\vec{D} = \varepsilon_0\, \vec{E} + \vec{P} = \varepsilon_r\, \varepsilon_0\, \vec{E} \tag{2.10}$$

By subtracting the effect of bound charges on the dielectric from the total electric field $\vec{E}$, the effect from free charges can be described as a function of the applied electric field across the dielectric. This is particularly useful to delineate the behavior of a dielectric medium in the presence of an external electric field.

Another important concept to consider about capacitors is that the charging and discharging characteristics do not change when operating either in direct or alternating current. However, this characteristic of the medium's dielectric properties affects the time constant of the material, which in turn affects the dielectric medium's response to the flow of electric current. This particular response is known as capacitive reactance, where the time constant is a way to describe the time it takes for charges within a medium to relax or approach electrostatic equilibrium (Eq. 2.11):

$$\tau = \frac{\varepsilon}{\sigma} \tag{2.11}$$

Materials with large time constants take a longer time for charges to approach electrostatic equilibrium, while those materials with a smaller time constants require a shorter duration. Interestingly, but not surprisingly, the time constant of a medium is frequency dependent and will change as the frequency of the applied alternating electric current changes. Equation 2.12 is the standard solution of a first-order homogeneous differential equation describing the discharge of a capacitor [19, 20]:

$$V(t) = V_0\, e^{-\frac{\sigma}{\varepsilon}t} \infty \tag{2.12}$$

For the purpose of exploring the differences of various tissue types within the brain, we consider a solved patient brain dataset with the respective dielectric properties applied, shown in Fig. 2.5A, exposed to a 200 kHz wave as the TTFields are programmed to emit through the arrays. After applying the appropriate dielectric properties of the various segmented tissues in the head, the model is solved. The cerebrospinal fluid (CSF) is mostly aqueous, mixed in with a variety of proteins and salts as it serves as a conduit between the central nervous system and the brain. Gray matter is composed mostly of lipids, behaving electrically more like an insulator or a material with a larger dielectric constant relative to CSF. Since the CSF in this

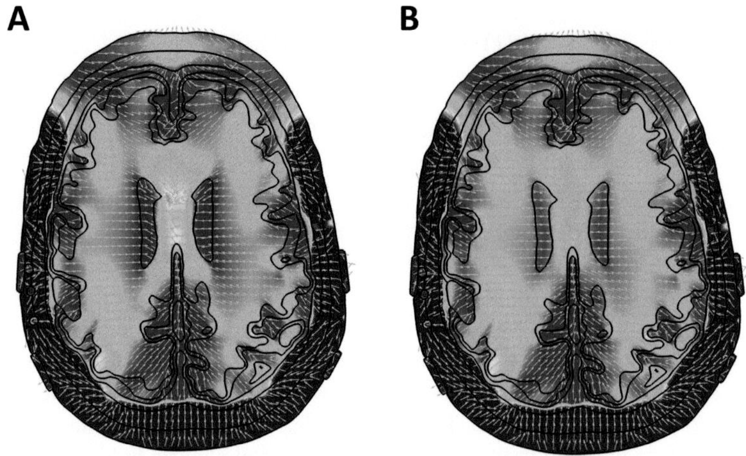


**Fig. 2.5** The effect of the highly conductive CSF compared to surrounding gray matter tissue with lower conductivity causes changes to the electric field distribution in the brain. (**A**) The electric field in the region between the bilateral ventricles, which are filled with CSF, experiences a higher intensity due to the relatively large conductivity difference compared between CSF and gray matter. (**B**) The electric field in the region between the bilateral ventricles when gray matter dielectric properties are applied to the bilateral ventricles evens out the differences in conductivity as in **A** and thus the field intensity is reduced. Note that the white vectors that overlay both maps, representing the direction of the electric field, are essentially pointing in the same direction and the magnitude of the electric fields is different between the two cases. *CSF* cerebrospinal fluid

example is more conductive than the block of gray matter in between, it would serve as the conductive terminals of a capacitor, while the gray matter in between would serve as the dielectric medium. The accepted isotropic electric conductivity of CSF and gray matter at 200 kHz is about 2 S/m and 0.141 S/m, respectively, while the accepted relative permittivity for CSF and gray matter at the same frequency is about 109 and 2010, respectively [21]. It has been shown that conductivity plays a greater role than permittivity in altering the distribution of TTFields within the brain [9, 22, 23].

In a modified model of the same brain dataset as described in Fig. 2.5A, when the dielectric properties of the bilateral ventricles are replaced with the gray matter dielectric properties, it can be observed that the electric field distribution in the region between the bilateral ventricles is vastly different (Fig. 2.5B). By applying TTFields in both constructs simultaneously, the electric potential will rise to a fully charged state at a much faster rate when CSF in the bilateral ventricle acts as the dielectric medium of a capacitor compared with gray matter as the dielectric. Similarly, when the electric potential source is disconnected from both capacitors after being fully charged, the discharging of both capacitors will commence. Once again, the capacitor with the CSF as a dielectric medium will discharge, or approach electrostatic equilibrium, at a faster rate than the capacitor with the gray matter as the dielectric. This ability for a medium to charge and discharge can be expressed as capacitive reactance, which is the resistance to change in electric potential in a capacitor (Eq. 2.13), where $f$ is the frequency of the applied electric potential and $C$ is the capacitance:

$$\chi = \frac{1}{2\pi fC} \tag{2.13}$$

For a constant direct current, which does not vary with time, the frequency component is 0, and therefore reactance does not apply. However, when an alternating current is applied as the electric potential source, there exists a frequency component that affects the ability of a capacitor to hold and retain charges over a cycle. For instance, from the example described in Fig. 2.5, when an alternating current is applied across either capacitor at 200 kHz, the only term left in Eq. 2.13 that determines the opposition to change in electric potential is the capacitance, which is inversely proportional to the capacitive reactance. Likewise, a lower capacitance results in a higher capacitive reactance or greater opposition to change in electric potential. Therefore, since CSF is more conductive than gray matter, CSF cannot retain enough charge to reach full potential before the field collapses and changes polarity.

## Specific Absorption Rate in Tissue from Tumor Treating Fields

An important and relevant quantity to the discussion of TTFields is the specific absorption rate (SAR), which is the amount of power absorbed by a unit mass of tissue (Eq. 2.14), where $\sigma$ is the conductivity of the inquired tissue, $\vec{E}$ is the electric field, and $\rho$ is the physical density of tissue. Power is defined as the change in energy over time and since TTFields are applied continuously over a long period of time, it is appropriate to quantify the amount of energy deposited in tissue in terms of power. Similar to the energy per unit mass of tissue as deposited by ionizing radiation that is expressed as dose in gray or J/kg, the rate of energy or power deposited by TTFields can be expressed as SAR or in W/kg. In computer modeling of electric fields in the brain, the delineation of SAR may help determine the amount of energy deposited over time at the tumor or other intracranial regions of interest:

$$SAR = \frac{\sigma\left|\vec{E}\right|^2}{\rho} \tag{2.14}$$

## Conclusions

An understanding of the basic physics principles of electricity and magnetism is of utmost importance to appreciate and learn more about the biophysical interactions within the brain induced by external electric fields applied on the surface of the scalp. The fundamental principles that govern TTFields include Coulomb's law, Gauss' law, Ohm's law, and the law of continuity. Derivatives of these equations to account for time-varying TTFields are essential to accurately describe the alternating electric field distribution within the brain during every cycle. Brain tissues are essentially dielectric materials with different conductivity and relative permittivity properties that change the electric field distribution due to their respective capacitive reactance characteristics and thus these distributions are nonuniform. Since TTFields are applied continuously in the patient, a more appropriate physical quantity to describe the amount of energy absorbed in the tissue media may be expressed in terms of power. Therefore, the concept of SAR can be used to describe the amount of power absorbed in a unit mass of tissue over the prolonged period of treatment time. With the fundamental biophysical characteristics established, the nature of TTFields and its probability and types of interaction with different tissues, cells, and subcellular components are then better understood, leading to our ability to further improve and develop this technology to provide better treatment outcomes for patients with glioblastoma and other malignancies.

## References


1. Stupp R, Hegi ME, Mason WP, et al. Effects of radiotherapy with concomitant and adjuvant temozolomide versus radiotherapy alone on survival in glioblastoma in a randomized phase III study: 5-year analysis of the EORTC-NCIC trial. Lancet Oncol. 2009;10:459–66.
2. Stupp R, Wong ET, Kanner AA, et al. NovoTTF-100A versus physician's choice chemotherapy in recurrent glioblastoma: a randomized phase III trial of a novel treatment modality. Eur J Cancer. 2012;48:2192–202.
3. Wong ET, Lok E, Guatam S, Swanson KD. Dexamethasone exerts profound immunologic interference on treatment efficacy for recurrent glioblastoma. Br J Cancer. 2015;113:232–41.
4. Stupp R, Tallibert S, Kanner AA, et al. Maintenance therapy with tumor-treating fields plus temozolomide vs temozolomide alone for glioblastoma: a randomized clinical trial. JAMA. 2015;314:2535–43.
5. Vymazal J, Wong ET. Response patterns of recurrent glioblastomas treated with tumor-treating fields. Semin Oncol. 2014;41 Suppl 6:S14–24.
6. Wong ET, Lok E, Swanson KD, et al. Response assessment of NovoTTF-100A versus best physician's choice chemotherapy in recurrent glioblastoma. Cancer Med. 2015;4:383–91.
7. Kirson ED, Gurvich Z, Schneiderman R, et al. Disruption of cancer cell replication by alternating electric fields. Cancer Res. 2004;64:3288–95.
8. Gera N, Yang A, Holtzman TS, et al. Tumor treating fields perturb the localization of septins and cause aberrant mitotic exit. PLoS One. 2015;10:e0125269.
9. Lok E, Swanson KD, Wong ET. Tumor treating fields therapy device for glioblastoma: physics and clinical practice considerations. Expert Rev Med Devices. 2015;12:717–26.
10. Lok E, Hua V, Wong ET. Computed modeling of alternating electric fields therapy for recurrent glioblastoma. Cancer Med. 2015;4:1697–9.
11. Stinstra JG, Peters MJ. The volume conductor may act as a temporal filter on the ECG and EEG. Med Biol Eng Comput. 1998;36:711–6.
12. Nolte G, Bai O, Wheaton L, Mari Z, Vorbach S, Hallett M. Identifying true brain interaction from EEG data using the imaginary part of coherency. Clin Neurophysiol. 2004;115:2292–307.

13. Wagner T, Valero-Cabre A, Pascual-Leone A. Noninvasive human brain stimulation. Annu Rev Biomed Eng. 2007;9:527–65.
14. Baillet S, Mosher JC, Laehy RM. Electromagnetic brain mapping. IEEE Signal Processing Magazine 2001;Nov:14–30.
15. Darvas F, Pantazis D, Kucukaltun-Yildirim E, Leahy RM. Mapping human brain function with MEG and EEG: methods and validation. Neuroimage. 2004;23 Suppl 1:S289–99.
16. Butson CR, McIntyre CC. Tissue and electrode capacitance reduce neural activation volumes during deep brain stimulation. Clin Neurophysiol. 2005;116:2490–500.
17. De Moerloose J, Dawson TW, Stuchly MA. Application of the finite difference time domain algorithm to quasi-static field analysis. Radio Sci. 1997;32:329–41.
18. Gabriel S, Lau RW, Gabriel C. The dielectric properties of biological tissues: III. Parametric models for the dielectric spectrum of tissues. Phys Med Biol. 1996;41:2271–93.
19. Reitz JR, Milford FJ, Christy RW. Foundations of electromagnetic theory. 4th ed. Reading: Addison-Wesley; 1993.
20. Griffith DJ. Introduction to electrodynamics. 3rd ed. Upper Saddle River: Prentice-Hall; 1999.
21. Hasgall PA, Di Gennaro F, Baumgartner C, et al. IT'IS Database for thermal and electromagnetic parameters of biological tissues, Version 2.6. 2015. www.itis.ethzch/database. Accessed 12 Aug 2014.
22. Miranda PC, Mekonnen A, Salvador R, Basser PJ. Predicting the electric field distribution in the brain for the treatment of glioblastoma. Phys Med Biol. 2014;59:4137–47.
23. Wenger C, Salvador R, Basser PJ, Miranda PC. The electric field distribution in the brain during TTFields therapy and its dependence on tissue dielectric properties and anatomy: a computational study. Phys Med Biol. 2015;60:7339–57.

# Chapter 3
# Biophysical Effects of Tumor Treating Fields

**Cornelia Wenger and Pedro C. Miranda**

Within the last decades, the effect of applied electric fields on biological cells has been extensively studied. At the cellular scale, different research groups concentrated their efforts on studying a variety of local effects from the electric field, such as the induced transmembrane voltage (TMV) under different stimulation conditions, as well as various single- and multiple-cell properties. The preliminary and most popular studies go back to H.P. Schwan and colleagues who not only analytically described the steady-state TMV induced in spherical cells [1], but also clarified mechanisms responsible for electrical properties of tissues and cell suspensions [2]. These insights were used to estimate the dielectric properties of cells and tissues allowing, for example, impedance measurements to differentiate normal and cancerous tissues [3]. Alongside, possible cell manipulation procedures employing electric fields have been investigated; that is, it was observed that cells may respond to AC polarization by orienting, deforming, moving, or rotating in a frequency-dependent manner [4, 5]. These investigations are applied for manipulation, trapping, separation, or sorting of biological cells or colloidal particles [4, 5].

Cellular scale observations can be translated into medical treatments and applications. The well-known techniques for nerve, muscle, and heart stimulation use DC pulses or very-low-frequency AC fields [6]. This relies on the fact that for frequencies below about 1 kHz, the excitable tissues can be stimulated through membrane depolarization. When the frequency increases, the response of the biological cell membranes is too slow to respond to high-frequency depolarization and thus becomes refractory to further stimulation. On the other hand, effects induced by very-high-

C. Wenger, Dr.techn. (✉) • P.C. Miranda, Ph.D.
Institute of Biophysics and Biomedical Engineering, Faculdade de Ciências, Universidade de Lisboa, 1749-016 Lisboa, Portugal
e-mail: cwenger@fc.ul.pt



E.T. Wong (ed.), *Alternating Electric Fields Therapy in Oncology*,
DOI 10.1007/978-3-319-30576-9_3

frequency fields range from heating to membrane disruption, electroporation, and cell death, depending on the field strength [5]. Commonly used medical treatments that utilize fields with frequencies in the high MHz or GHz range are diathermy and radiofrequency tumor ablation. In summary, most of the investigation of the response of cells to AC electromagnetic fields has focused on the low-frequency (<10 kHz) or high-frequency ranges (MHz or GHz). Intermediate-frequency AC electric fields in the kHz to MHz region were long thought to have no meaningful biological effect and are just currently being investigated in more detail [7–12].

One technique that makes use of this intermediate-frequency range is a relatively new modality for cancer treatment termed Tumor Treating Fields (TTFields). This method relies on low-intensity, between 1 and 3 V/cm, and intermediate-frequency, between 100 and 300 kHz, alternating electric fields that have been shown *in vitro* and *in vivo* to destroy selectively dividing cells that are undergoing mitosis and cytokinesis [7, 13–15]. One assumed mechanism of action is an anti-microtubule effect whereby tubulin subunits are forced to align with the applied field, perturbing the formation of functional mitotic spindles that are essential for the completion of mitosis. A second possible mechanism of action relates to a dielectrophoretic (DEP) effect since the cellular morphology during cytokinesis gives rise to a non-uniform intracellular electric field, with a high gradient at the furrow between the dividing cells exerting forces on polar macromolecules and organelles. Preclinical data demonstrated mitotic arrest, and subsequent apoptosis of different cancer cell lines, as well as structural disruption associated with violent membrane blebbing [7]. TTFields treatment spares quiescent cells and specifically targets cancer cells undergoing mitosis, with a particular optimal frequency of largest inhibitory effect for each cell line tested [7, 13, 16].

TTFields are currently used to treat glioblastoma multiforme (GBM) patients. The Optune® system is a medical device that was developed to deliver the TTFields to the brain via transducer arrays placed on the patient's scalp. Following the mentioned *in vitro* experiments, these transducers deliver alternating electric fields of 200 kHz in two perpendicular directions. Optune® was approved for the treatment of recurrent GBM by the U.S. Food and Drug Administration in 2011 [17]. In October 2015, TTFields in combination with temozolomide was also approved for newly diagnosed GBM patients [18, 19].

## Computational Cell Models

Although the electric behavior of simple cell morphologies like spheres or ellipsoids can be described analytically, more complex and realistic shapes can only be investigated with the help of computational models. There already exist some studies that specifically investigate the electric field distribution within the quiescent and the dividing cell induced by alternating, intermediate-frequency, low-intensity fields [8, 9, 12]. In all of these studies, the finite element method (FEM) is used to

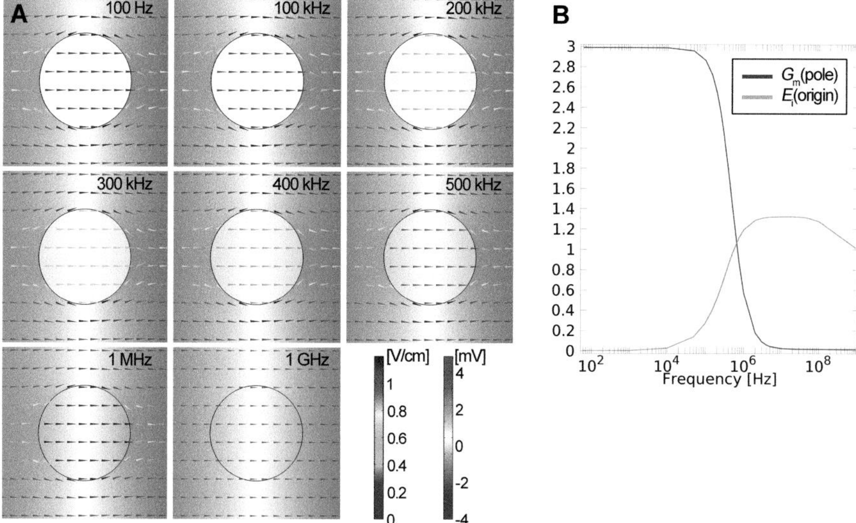


**Fig. 3.1** Frequency effect of the electric field on mitotic cell. (**A**) The electric field is represented by *arrows* with corresponding rainbow color scale (V/cm). Surface plots of the electric potential are also presented (mV). Different frequencies have been selected. (**B**) Line plots of the membrane field gain at the cell's pole (*blue*) and the intracellular electric field strength $E_i$ at the origin as a function of frequency. Adapted from Wenger et al. [12].

solve for the electric potential in and around single cells, enabling the calculation of the TMV, i.e., $U_m = \varphi_i - \varphi_e$, and the electric field distribution.

Since the cell rounds up during mitosis [20, 21], it can be represented as a sphere with a very thin membrane with a thickness $d_m$ which separates the intracellular from the extracellular space (Fig. 3.1A). Thus, three domains are distinguished which possess different dielectric properties, i.e., specific values of the electric conductivity $\sigma$ and the relative permittivity $\varepsilon$ (Table 3.1).

## The Effect of Frequency on the Electric Field During Metaphase

If an alternating electric field of magnitude $E_e$ is applied to the extracellular space, the magnitude of the resulting electric fields in the membrane, $E_m$, and the intracellular space, $E_i$, are frequency dependent. Furthermore, the field inside a homogeneous spherical cell placed in a uniform applied field is also uniform (Fig. 3.1A). In order to examine the frequency dependency of the induced fields some authors plot the (normalized) potential at the cell's pole against frequency, e.g., [22–24]. Others discuss the membrane field gain $G_m$, which reflects the frequency-dependent

**Table 3.1** Standard, minimum (min), and maximum (max) values of geometric and dielectric properties.

| | Unit | Min | Standard | Max | |
|---|---|---|---|---|---|
| $r_{cell}$ | [μm] | 4 | 10 | 15 | Cell radius |
| $d_m$ | [nm] | – | 5 | – | Membrane diameter |
| $\sigma_i$ | [S/m] | 0.1 | 0.3 | 0.9 | Intracellular electric conductivity |
| $\sigma_e$ | [S/m] | 0.9 | 1.2 | 1.2 | Extracellular electric conductivity |
| $\sigma_m$ | [S/m] | $3\times10^{-7}$ | $3\times10^{-7}$ | $5\times10^{-5}$ | Membrane electric conductivity |
| $\varepsilon_i$ | | 60 | 72.3 | 80 | Intracellular relative permittivity |
| $\varepsilon_e$ | | 60 | 72.3 | 80 | Extracellular relative permittivity |
| $\varepsilon_m$ | | 2.5 | 5 | 7.5 | Membrane relative permittivity |

amplification of the applied field in the membrane, and is defined as $G_m(\omega) = \frac{E_m(\omega)}{E_e}$, where $\omega$ is the angular frequency [25, 26]. Since the cell membrane is assumed homogenous, the induced membrane electric field can be expressed as $E_m(\omega) = \frac{U_m(\omega)}{d_m}$, and therefore $G_m(\omega) = \frac{U_m(\omega)}{d_m E_e}$.

The values of $G_m$ and thus also $E_i$ certainly change for different frequencies of the applied electric field (Fig. 3.1B). For very low frequencies below about 1 kHz, $G_m$ is constant and high, resulting in almost zero intracellular field strength $E_i$. As the frequency increases the TMV decreases, the amplification of the membrane electric field is reduced, and the electric field "invades" the cell, increasing its strength $E_i$. This can be observed in Fig. 3.1B by the descent of the blue $G_m$ curve and the increase of the green $E_i$ curve. The TMV is basically independent of frequency until the angular frequency $\omega = 2\pi f$ becomes comparable with the reciprocal of the time constant:

$$\tau = \frac{r_{cell} \cdot \frac{\varepsilon_m}{d_m}}{\frac{2\sigma_e \sigma_i}{2\sigma_e + \sigma_i} + \frac{r_{cell}}{d_m}\sigma_m}. \tag{3.1}$$

As has been stated (Eq. 3.1), the limit for low-frequency potential for typical cell sizes ranges from the upper kHz to the lower MHz range. With the standard parameters given in Table 3.1, this breakpoint frequency is 480 kHz, which is exactly the point where the blue line in Fig. 3.1 starts to descend. In the low-MHz region, when this line drops below $G_m = 1$, which marks the region where $E_m < E_e$, the electric field inside the cell becomes higher than the applied field in the extracellular space. Zero values of the field gain $G_m$ signify total uniformity in all domains, with the electric fields equalized to the value of the excitation field, i.e., $E_m = E_i = E_e$.

This behavior is also illustrated in the first column in Fig. 3.1A. Up to 100 kHz the electric field inside the cell, in blue cones, is lower than the field in the extracellular space. As the frequency approaches the breakpoint the intracellular electric field strength starts to increase. At 500 kHz the field strengths inside and outside the cell become equal, and are plotted in orange cones. At slightly higher frequencies, the membrane field gain becomes lower than 1 and the field inside the cell, now in red, becomes higher than that in the outside. The last plot at the bottom right illustrates the convergence to the excitation intensity.

## The Effect of Dielectric Properties on the Electric Field During Metaphase

The assumed dielectric properties of the biological media vary between publications. Many computational studies [22, 25, 27–29] concerning similar investigations adopt values for the conductivity and relative permittivity from previous studies [23, 30, 31]. Those values were taken from investigations on yeast cells [32], erythroleukemia cells [33], and T and B lymphocytes [34]. Yet, these parameters are also used for studying neurons [35, 36]. Furthermore, different values may also be expected for glial cells [37–41] and pronounced differences exist between the electrical properties of some cancerous and non-cancerous tissues [5]. Thus, we systematically tested the effect of changing the dielectric properties on the intracellular field strength [8, 12], for the range of values presented in Table 3.1. Figure 3.2 summarizes the most important consequences in the observed electric behavior and plots the intracellular field strength $E_i$ as function of frequency. Increasing $E_i$ is predicted for increasing $\sigma_m$ without shifting significantly the frequency at which $E_i$ increases most rapidly (Fig. 3.2A). When $\varepsilon_m$ is increased, $E_i$ also increases with an earlier and faster growth for higher $\varepsilon_m$ values (Fig. 3.2B). Decreasing $E_i$ is predicted for increasing $\sigma_i$ with an earlier and faster growth for lower $\sigma_i$ values (Fig. 3.2C). Changes in $\sigma_e$, $\varepsilon_e$, and $\varepsilon_i$ affect $E_i$ only at very high frequencies (Fig. 3.2D).

In summary, the simulations with the spherical metaphase cell predict a uniform intracellular field with nonzero $E_i$. Depending on cell properties, the frequency window of the predicted transition range might be shifted.

## The Effect of Cell Shape on the Electric Field During Telophase

During telophase the two dividing sister cells have elliptical cell shape [20, 21]. The simulations we performed [8, 12] assume three different stages of cytokinesis; that is, two ellipsoids with major radii of 10 μm and minor radii of 7 μm

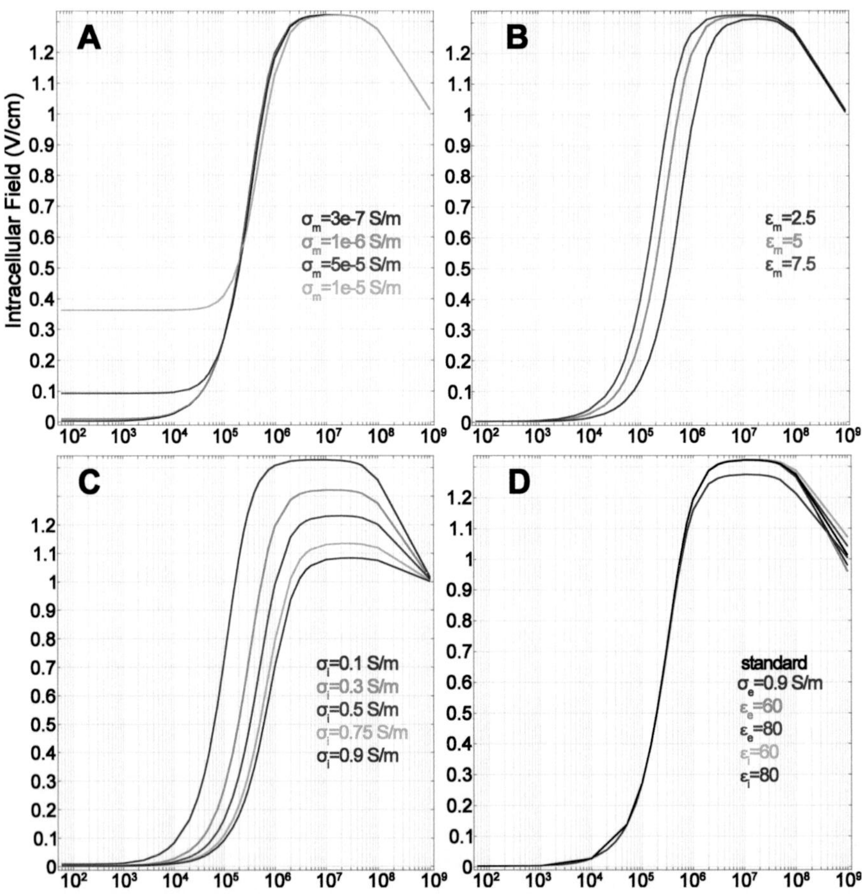


**Fig. 3.2** The intracellular field strength $E_i$ at the center of the cell as a function of frequency for varying $\sigma_m$ (**A**), $\varepsilon_m$ (**B**), $\sigma_i$ (**C**), and in $\sigma_e$, $\varepsilon_e$, and $\varepsilon_i$ (**D**). Adapted from Wenger et al. [12].

(minor radius is always 70 % of the major radius) are pulled apart by increasing the distance between the cell centers by 50 %, 90 %, and 99 % of the cell major diameter, respectively (Fig. 3.3). In contrast to what was observed in the spherical metaphase cell, the intracellular electric field is non-uniform and converges towards the cleavage plane separating the two sister cells. Figure 3.3 shows a surface plot of electric field displayed with fixed color range with selected frequencies plotted in rows and cytokinesis stages in columns. Again $E_i$ is almost zero at low frequencies, but field non-uniformity becomes apparent in the low-kHz range. This is particularly visible for later stages of cytokinesis (third and fourth columns in Fig. 3.3) with corresponding maximum $E_i$ values that are much higher than the applied field of 1 V/cm.

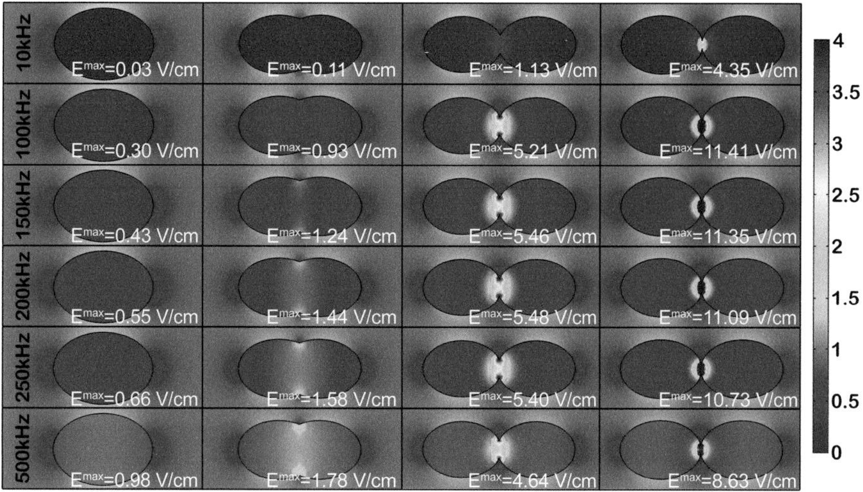


**Fig. 3.3** Electric field distribution for selected frequencies (*rows*) and different stages of cytokinesis (*columns*). Adapted from Wenger et al. [12].

The right column of Fig. 3.3 with almost separated sister cells shows the most pronounced and spatially confined electric field at the furrow, which is present even for a low 10 kHz stimulation frequency. At higher frequencies, the non-uniformity close to the furrow decreases as the field strength further increases throughout the cell. The highest maximum value of $E_i$ of 11.41 V/cm is predicted for stimulation at 100 kHz, in the last stage of cytokinesis. The furrow between the cells is longer in an earlier stage of cytokinesis depicted in the third column, and the highest maximum value of $E_i$, 5.48 V/cm, is reached at 200 kHz.

A non-uniform electric field induces unidirectional DEP forces. This DEP force leads to the motion of polarizable particles as a result of the interaction of a non-uniform electric field $\boldsymbol{E}$ with their induced dipole moment $p$, i.e., $\boldsymbol{F} = p \cdot \nabla \boldsymbol{E}$ [42], and it is proportional to the square of the gradient of the electric field, i.e., $|\boldsymbol{F}| \propto \left|\nabla|\boldsymbol{E}|^2\right|$ [43, 44]. The term $\left|\nabla|\boldsymbol{E}|^2\right|$ is referred to as the DEP force component, and has units of $V^2/m^3$. In analogy with the observed $E_i$ peaks, also the DEP force component shows stage-specific peak frequencies. This is displayed in Fig. 3.4B where the normalized DEP force component is plotted as function of frequency for the three cytokinesis stages. Well-defined peak frequencies are observed at 450 kHz, 175 kHz, and 125 kHz for stage 1 (orange), stage 2 (green), and stage 3 (blue), respectively. Thus, the peak frequency is decreasing for later stages of cytokinesis, but with increasing absolute force component values.

The reported peak frequency values correspond well with the reported frequency dependence of TTFields [7, 13]. Furthermore the dose dependency of TTFields [7], which relates to the fact that the inhibitory effect of TTFields increases rapidly with

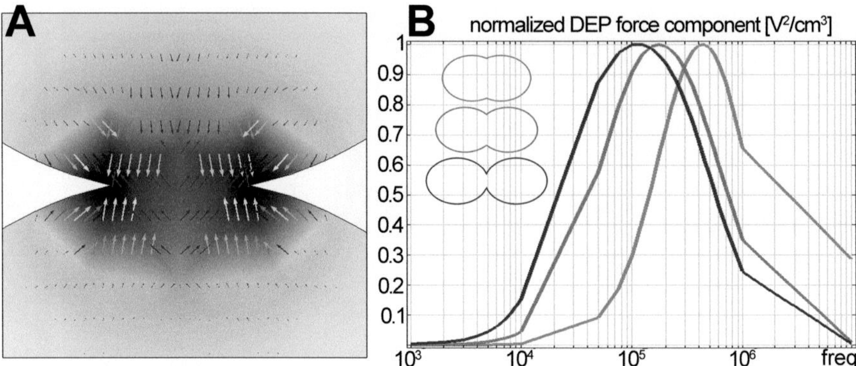


**Fig. 3.4** DEP forces on a cell during cytokinesis. (**A**) Close-up of the furrow region and the DEP force component plotted as *arrows*. (**B**) The normalized DEP force component for the three stages of cytokinesis. Adapted from Wenger et al. [12].

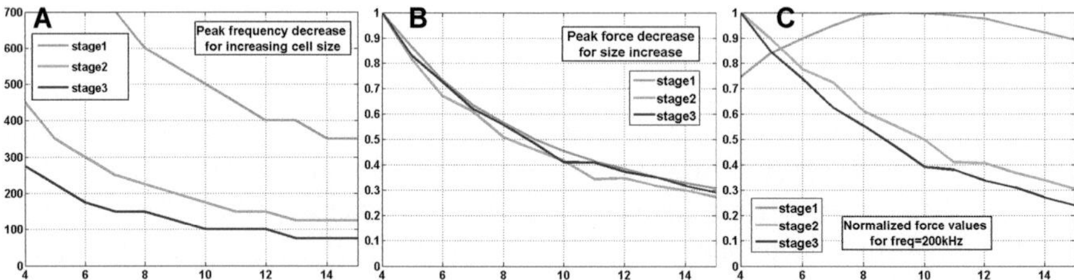


**Fig. 3.5** Cellular characteristics that influence DEP forces. (**A**) The peak frequency (kHz) of maximal DEP force component as a function of cell radius (μm) for the three stages of cytokinesis. (**B**) Normalized maximal peak force values, plotted as functions of cell radius. (**C**) The normalized DEP force component values at 200 kHz for the three stages.

increasing applied field strength, was confirmed by this computational modeling approach [8, 12]. One additional experimentally observed effect was that the optimal frequency for inhibitory effect of TTFields is inversely related to cell size [7, 13], and increased cell volume is seen in almost all cell lines treated with TTFields [45]. Again computational modeling predicted similar results, by repeating the simulations with dividing cells whose major radius ranges from 4 to 15 μm. Figure 3.5A shows that the peak frequencies (in kHz) of the DEP force component decrease and then level off with increasing cell radius (in μm). The corresponding maximum values of the DEP force component also decrease for increasing cell size, but the normalized decay rate is the same for all cytokinesis stages (Fig. 3.5B). Consequently, for a constant 200 kHz TTFields frequency, smaller cells in late cytokinesis are exposed to higher force (Fig. 3.5C). This indicates that a larger cell might be less affected by the field.

## Conclusion

This comprehensive description serves as a first approach to further elucidate the details behind the mechanisms of action of TTFields, and more generally to provide a deeper understanding of the electric field distribution within cells under the influence of alternating electric fields. It also illustrates how computational modeling can be used to systematically investigate the effect of changes in cell physical properties, shape, and size on the intracellular electric field. Future insights into the biophysical effects of alternating electric fields may be gained through computational modeling at the subcellular level or at the level of cell assemblies.

## References

1. Grosse C, Schwan HP. Cellular membrane potentials induced by alternating fields. Biophys J . 1992;63(6):1632–42.
2. Schwan HP. Mechanisms responsible for electrical properties of tissues and cell suspensions. Med Prog Technol. 1993-1994;19(4):163–5.
3. Laufer S, Ivorra A, Reuter VE, Rubinsky B, Solomon SB. Electrical impedance characterization of normal and cancerous human hepatic tissue. Physiol Meas. 2010;31(7):995–1009.
4. Gimsa J. A comprehensive approach to electro-orientation, electrodeformation, dielectrophoresis, and electrorotation of ellipsoidal particles and biological cells. Bioelectrochemistry. 2001;54(1):23–31.
5. Markx GH. The use of electric fields in tissue engineering: a review. Organogenesis. 2008;4(1):11–7.
6. Malmivuo J, Plonsey R. Bioelectromagnetism. New York: Oxford University Press; 1995.
7. Kirson ED, Gurvich Z, Schneiderman R, Dekel E, Itzhaki A, Wasserman Y, et al. Disruption of cancer cell replication by alternating electric fields. Cancer Res. 2004;64(9):3288–95.
8. Wenger C, Miranda PC, Salvador R, Basser PJ. Investigating the mechanisms of action of tumor treating fields: a computational modeling study. Neuro-Oncol. 2014;16 Suppl 5:v216.
9. Taghian T, Narmoneva DA, Kogan AB. Modulation of cell function by electric field: a high-resolution analysis. J R Soc Interface. 2015;12(107):pii: 20150153.
10. Liang J, Mok AW, Zhu Y, Shi J. Resonance versus linear responses to alternating electric fields induce mechanistically distinct mammalian cell death. Bioelectrochemistry. 2013;94:61–8.
11. Uppalapati M, Huang Y-M, Jackson TN, Hancock WO. Microtubule alignment and manipulation using AC electrokinetics. Small. 2008;4(9):1371–81.
12. Wenger C, Giladi M, Bomzon Z, Salvador R, Basser PJ, Miranda PC. Modeling Tumor Treating Fields (TTFields) application in single cells during metaphase and telophase. Engineering in Medicine and Biology Society (EMBC), 2015. 37th Annual International Conference of the IEEE, 2015. p. 6892–5.
13. Kirson ED, Dbalý V, Tovarys F, Vymazal J, Soustiel JF, Itzhaki A, et al. Alternating electric fields arrest cell proliferation in animal tumor models and human brain tumors. Proc Natl Acad Sci U S A. 2007;104(24):10152–7.
14. Gera N, Yang A, Holtzman TS, Lee SX, Wong ET, Swanson KD. Tumor treating fields perturbs the localization of septins and cause aberrant mitotic exit. PLoS One. 2015;10:e0125269.
15. Giladi M, Schneiderman RS, Voloshin T, Porat Y, Munster M, Blat R, et al. Mitotic spindle disruption by alternating electric fields leads to improper chromosome segregation and mitotic catastrophe in cancer cells. Sci Rep 2015;5:18046.

16. Giladi M, Porat Y, Blatt A, Wasserman Y, Kirson ED, Dekel E, et al. Microbial growth inhibition by alternating electric fields. Antimicrob Agents Chemother. 2008;52(10):3517–22.
17. Stupp R, Wong ET, Kanner AA, Steinberg D, Engelhard H, Heidecke V, et al. NovoTTF-100A versus physician's choice chemotherapy in recurrent glioblastoma: a randomised phase III trial of a novel treatment modality. Eur J Cancer. 2012;48(14):2192–202.
18. Stupp R, Taillibert S, Kanner AA, Kesari S, Steinberg DM, Toms SA, et al. Maintenance therapy with tumor-treating fields plus temozolomide vs temozolomide alone for glioblastoma: a randomized clinical trial. JAMA. 2015;314:2535-43.
19. http://www.fda.gov/NewsEvents/Newsroom/PressAnnouncements/ucm465744.htm
20. Boucrot E, Kirchhausen T. Mammalian cells change volume during mitosis. PLoS One. 2008;3(1):1477.
21. Habela CW, Sontheimer H. Cytoplasmic volume condensation is an integral part of mitosis. Cell Cycle. 2007;6(13):1613–20.
22. Stewart DA, Gowrishankar TR, Smith KC, Weaver JC. Cylindrical cell membranes in uniform applied electric fields: validation of a transport lattice method. IEEE Trans Biomed Eng. 2005;52(10):1643–53.
23. Kotnik T, Miklavčič D. Theoretical evaluation of voltage inducement on internal membranes of biological cells exposed to electric fields. Biophys J. 2006;90(2):480–91.
24. Pavlin M, Miklavčič D. The effective conductivity and the induced transmembrane potential in dense cell system exposed to DC and AC electric fields. IEEE Trans Plasma Sci. 2009;37(1):99–106.
25. Gowrishankar TR, Weaver JC. An approach to electrical modeling of single and multiple cells. Proc Natl Acad Sci U S A. 2003;100(6):3203–8.
26. Kotnik T, Miklavčič D. Analytical description of transmembrane voltage induced by electric fields on spheroidal cells. Biophys J. 2000;79(2):670–9.
27. Gowrishankar TR, Stewart DA, Weaver JC. Model of a confined spherical cell in uniform and heterogeneous applied electric fields. Bioelectrochemistry. 2006;68(2):181–90.
28. Vajrala V, Claycomb JR, Sanabria H, Miller JH. Effects of oscillatory electric fields on internal membranes: an analytical model. Biophys J. 2008;94(6):2043–52.
29. Tiwari PK, Kang SK, Kim GJ, Choi J, Mohamed A-AH, Lee JK. Modeling of nanoparticle-mediated electric field enhancement inside biological cells exposed to AC electric fields. Jpn J Appl Phys. 2009;48(8):087001.
30. Kotnik T, Bobanović F, Miklavčič D. Sensitivity of transmembrane voltage induced by applied fields—a theoretical analysis. Bioelectrochem Bioenerg. 1997;43(43):285–91.
31. Kotnik T, Miklavčič D. Second-order model of membrane electric field induced by alternating external electric fields. IEEE Trans Biomed Eng. 2000;47(8):1074–81.
32. Hölzel R, Lamprecht I. Dielectric properties of yeast cells as determined by electrorotation. Biochim Biophys Acta. 1992;1104(1):195–200.
33. Gascoyne PR, Pethig R, Burt JP, Becker FF. Membrane changes accompanying the induced differentiation of Friend murine erythroleukemia cells studied by dielectrophoresis. Biochim Biophys Acta. 1993;1149(1):119–26.
34. Hu X, Arnold WM, Zimmermann U. Alterations in the electrical properties of T and B lymphocyte membranes induced by mitogenic stimulation. Activation monitored by electrorotation of single cells. Biochim Biophys Acta. 1990;1021(2):191–200.
35. Ye H, Cotic M, Kang EE, Fehlings MG, Carlen PL. Transmembrane potential induced on the internal organelle by a time-varying magnetic field: a model study. J Neuroeng Rehabil. 2010;7:12.
36. Ye H, Cotic M, Fehlings MG, Carlen PL. Influence of cellular properties on the electric field distribution around a single cell. Prog Electromagn Res B. 2012;39:141–61.
37. Hild W, Tasaki I. Morphological and physiological properties of neurons and glial cells in tissue culture. J Neurophysiol. 1962;25:277–304.
38. Trachtenberg MC, Kornblith PL, Häuptli J. Biophysical properties of cultured human glial cells. Brain Res. 1972;38:279–98.
39. Somjen GG. Electrophysiology of neuroglia. Annu Rev Physiol. 1975;37(171):163–90.

40. Bédard C, Kröger H, Destexhe A. Modeling extracellular field potentials and the frequency-filtering properties of extracellular space. Biophys J. 2004;86(3):1829–42.
41. Hille B. Ionic channels of excitable membranes. 2nd ed. Sunderland, MA: Sinauer Associates Inc., 1992.
42. Pohl HA. Dielectrophoresis. Cambridge, UK: Cambridge University Press, 1978.
43. Sun T, Morgan H, Green N. Analytical solutions of ac electrokinetics in interdigitated electrode arrays: electric field, dielectrophoretic and traveling-wave dielectrophoretic forces. Phys Rev E. 2007;76(4):046610.
44. Jones TB. Basic theory of dielectrophoresis and electrorotation. Eng Med Biol Mag IEEE. 2003;22(6):33–42.
45. Giladi M, Schneiderman RS, Porat Y, Munster M, Itzhaki A, Mordechovich D, et al. Mitotic disruption and reduced clonogenicity of pancreatic cancer cells in vitro and in vivo by tumor treating fields. Pancreatology. 2014;14(1):54–63.

# Chapter 4
# Computer Simulation of Tumor Treating Fields

**Edwin Lok, Eric T. Wong, and Erno Sajo**

Tumor Treating Fields (TTFields) use frequency-tuned alternating electric fields at 200 kHz that disrupt tumor cells as they undergo mitosis. The targets of these fields are proteins such as α/β tubulin and septin that have high dipole moments. In the patient, TTFields are applied on the scalp by two pairs of orthogonally positioned transducer arrays. Because the energy delivered by TTFields is relatively low, the electric field is spatially distorted by variations in the local conductivity and relative permittivity of tissues and fluid cavities within the brain. This is in contradistinction to ionizing radiation used in external beam radiation therapy, in which high-energy beams at the higher frequency end of the electromagnetic spectrum are delivered to tissues, which are amenable to dosimetry delineation of the tumor target. In both cases significant computer resources are required for treatment planning and verification. While in external beam radiation therapy the challenge is represented by difficulties in determining the tissue cross sections and the presence of heterogeneous geometries, leading to complex radiation transport simulations based on a priori diagnostic imaging information, the nature of the problem in TTFields therapy is different. Instead of

E. Lok, M.S. (✉)
Division of Neuro-Oncology, Department of Neurology, Beth Israel Deaconess Medical Center, Boston, MA 02215, USA
e-mail: elok@bidmc.harvard.edu

E.T. Wong, M.D.
Division of Neuro-Oncology, Department of Neurology, Beth Israel Deaconess Medical Center, Boston, MA, USA

Department of Physics, University of Massachusetts in Lowell, Lowell, MA 01854, USA

E. Sajo, Ph.D.
Department of Physics, University of Massachusetts Lowell, Lowell, MA 01854, USA

 
E.T. Wong (ed.), *Alternating Electric Fields Therapy in Oncology*,
DOI 10.1007/978-3-319-30576-9_4

having to solve the coupled charged particle-photon linear Boltzmann equation, solutions to the coupled Maxwell equations are needed to visualize directly how TTFields infiltrate the tumor and the surrounding brain tissues. The methods of computation, such as finite element analysis, and root-finding algorithms (e.g., Newton-Raphson method), rely on computer software like Mimics® (Materialize, Belgium) or ScanIP® (Simpleware, UK) and COMSOL Multiphysics® (COMSOL Burlington, Massachusetts, USA) for imaging processing and simulation.

## Energy Delivery via Tumor Treating Fields Versus Ionizing Radiation

TTFields and ionizing radiation deliver energies using significantly different parts of the electromagnetic spectrum. The frequency at which TTFields operate is in the kilohertz or $10^3$ cycles/seconds range with a wavelength of about ten football fields long, and the amount of energy delivered is quantified in terms of power per unit mass (W/kg) or energy per unit time per unit mass (J/s/kg), which is the dose rate. In contrast, X-rays and gamma rays operate in the exahertz or $10^{19}$ cycles/seconds range with a wavelength smaller than the diameter of a hydrogen atom, and the energy delivered over a specific time interval is measured in terms of the dose with units of J/kg or Gy. While most external beam radiation therapy uses ionizing radiation with beam-on time of only a few minutes per fraction, the duration of TTFields therapy is orders of magnitude longer. Therefore, on a per unit time basis, TTFields deliver a lower amount of energy to the target tissue than ionizing radiation. Nevertheless, they both damage actively dividing tumor cells and effect downstream anticancer responses. Apart from this similarity, the two types of therapies diverge in their mechanisms of action.

According to the current theory of radiobiology, irreparable radiation injury of cells leads to mitotic death. Therefore, ionizing radiation damages tumors more effectively than normal tissues because tumor cells actively divide and undergo the mitotic process more often than normal cells. There are two main mechanisms of damage, direct and indirect actions, which form the basis for ionizing radiation's anticancer efficacy. In the case of direct action the incident radiation directly ionizes subcellular targets like DNA causing breaks in chemical bonds, which in turn can lead to single- and double-strand DNA breaks (SSB and DSB) resulting in cell death if not repaired [1–4]. Indirect action is mediated by reactive molecular species such as solvated electrons and free radicals, which are generated via the radiolysis of water. They can also cause SSB and DSB in the DNA and other types of damage to cellular organelles within the tumor [5, 6]. Unfortunately, the effects of radiation cannot be confined to the tumor, and limited damage to adjacent normal tissue is almost inevitable despite the ever-increasing sophistication of treatment planning and delivery. Therefore, radiation necrosis, radiation-induced encephalopathy, and radiation-induced myelopathy are some of the consequences of ionizing radiation's side effects in the central nervous system [7–9].

TTFields deliver energy into a given mass of tissue continuously and the alternating electric fields target specifically those subcellular components of the mitotic machinery that have high dipole moments. Two such components, namely α/β tubulin and septin that have respective dipole moments of 1660 and 2711 Debyes [10], have been observed to be disrupted by TTFields during the transition from metaphase to anaphase in dividing tumor cells, leading to downstream interference with chromosome segregation and cytokinesis [11, 12]. The treated tumor cells may not die immediately but may need to go through multiple rounds of division before they die of apoptosis or immunogenic cell death [13, 14]. However, no toxicities within the brain have been observed and the major adverse events appear to be dermatological in nature, manifesting as scalp irritation [15].

## Computational Physics and Simulation

Current methods of computational physics rely on a combination of (1) comprehensive understanding of the problem to be solved and the development of its mathematical model, (2) appropriate analytical and numerical methods and their combinations that implement an efficient approach to solving these problems, and (3) available computational hardware to perform the simulations. In an idealized situation, many physical behaviors can be modeled by the application of the fundamental laws of physics, alone or in combinations, and their solutions obtained analytically. However, in practice, most problems are too complex to be solved analytically and approximations are necessary both in the mathematical model and its solution. One of the methods in solving boundary value problems in partial differential equations, which is often used in TTFields modeling, is the finite element method (FEM). Early applications of FEM were first introduced in mechanical engineering, most notably in fluid dynamics by the aerospace industry during the 1950s and 1960s [16–19]. With the advent of faster digital computers, it has recently gained wide acceptance in other fields as well.

To visualize the electric field distribution within the brain delivered by the Optune® device, the computational procedures involve three essential steps: (1) segmenting various brain structures, (2) applying appropriate conditions and material properties, and (3) solving the coupled Maxwell equations using finite element analysis. First, patient image datasets, including MRI (T1, T2, and MP RAGE), CT, and PET, are typically acquired as DICOM formatted image files, which are then co-registered using post-acquisition processing software such as Mimics® or ScanIP®. Co-registration of various scanning techniques is essential in order to produce segmented structures of the various types of tissues and cavities within the brain, allowing for optimal visualization and high fidelity in processing anatomic structures that have low contrast (Fig. 4.1). For example, it is rather difficult to discern between white matter and gray matter in the brain on CT but they can be distinguished easier on MRI. Likewise, lymph nodes in the body that are infiltrated by tumors are much harder to detect on CT scans but are readily identified on PET due to the uptake of $^{18}$fluorodeoxyglucose by

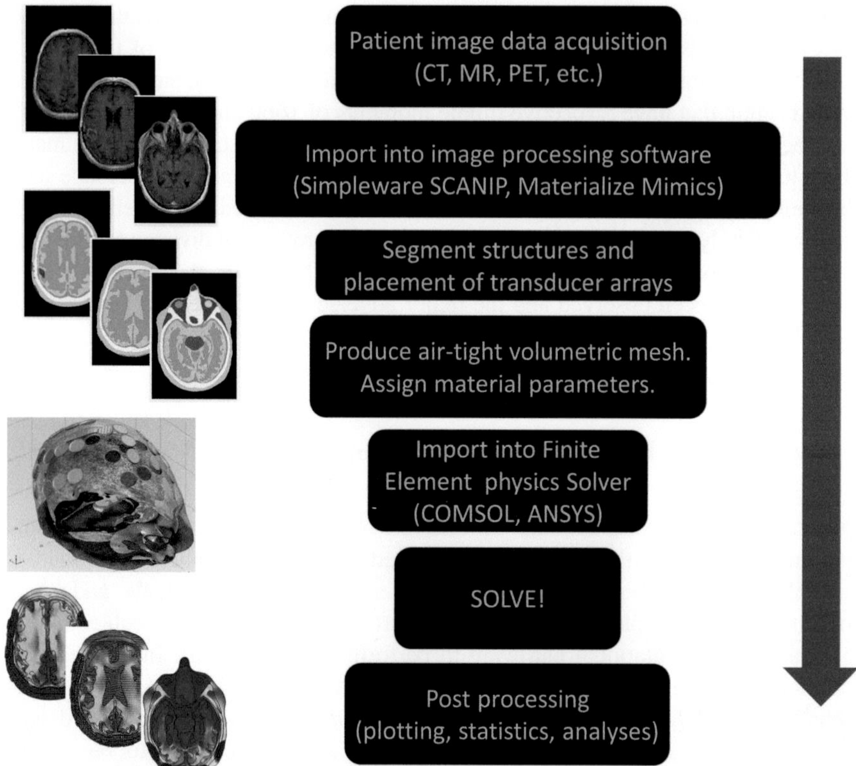


**Fig. 4.1** Workflow diagram for segmentation, co-registration, and computer simulation of electric field distribution within the brain

tumor cells. From these co-registered images, the main anatomic structures are segmented into separate masks. When all the structures have been completely segmented, including filling in "islands" and small cavities by a combination of manual and automated segmentation techniques, a completely filled 3-dimensional mesh is then generated based on the segmented volumes. This 3-dimensional mesh (Fig. 4.2) is then imported into a finite element solver such as the one from COMSOL Multiphysics® to solve the coupled Maxwell equations and produce a visualization of the electric field distribution in the human brain.

Although segmentation of various tissues and structures can be completed using a combination of automated features available in the image post-processing software, the results do not always turn out to be accurate or produced with high fidelity. As suggested in a study by Guo D. et al. [20], the digitized results from automated segmentation by statistical parametric mapping produce pixels in the FEM that do not optimally represent the true geometry and in the numerical solution of Maxwell's equations result in errors or singularities due to poor convergence. These non-convergent pixels (a.k.a. "dead" or "floating" pixels) require manual correction [20].

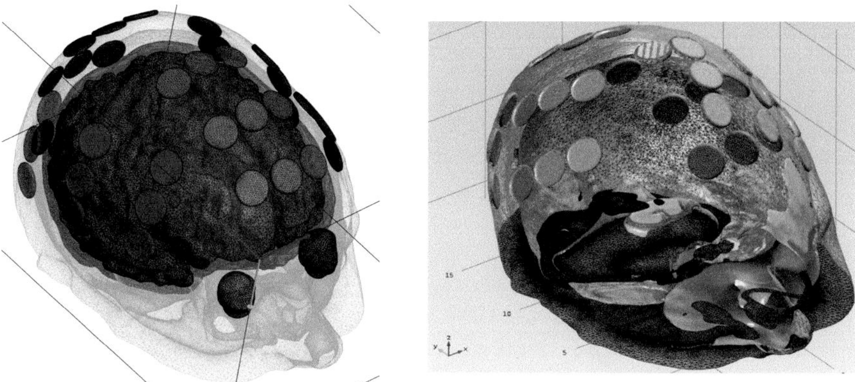

**Fig. 4.2** A 3-dimensional representation of human head generated based on segmented volumes before (left) and after (right) importation into a finite element solver

Although the presence of several non-convergent pixels may not necessarily change the computation of the electric field distribution in a significant way, one must strive to eliminate these errors in order to obtain the best possible representation. However, an even more important reason to eliminate the floating pixels is to reduce the chance of producing a singularity in the result due to the inability to produce a correct finite element representation of the geometry over the affected pixel, or producing a singularity-like result due to dramatic changes in physical parameters such as electric conductivity. Therefore, it is imperative not to disregard such errors while preparing the finite element mesh.

When the mesh has been imported into a finite element solver, physical parameters that represent the composition of the various segmented anatomical structures are applied to each structure along with initial and boundary conditions as well as input parameters for the computation. For instance, in order to solve for the electric field distribution throughout the brain from TTFields induced by the transducer arrays that are placed against the scalp as seen in Fig. 4.3, the electric conductivity and relative permittivity values are applied to each segmented volume in the mesh model. Initial conditions for these domains include an assumed initial electric potential = 0 or current density = 0, and the boundaries between all domains and elements are continuous. Input parameters may include the applied voltage or current from the transducer arrays following a standard sinusoidal waveform as described in Chapter 2.

## Newton-Raphson Method for Iterative Root Finding

The distribution of TTFields cannot be solved analytically and therefore numerical techniques must be used to approximate the solution. One of the most basic techniques of numerically finding the roots of a set of coupled equations that otherwise

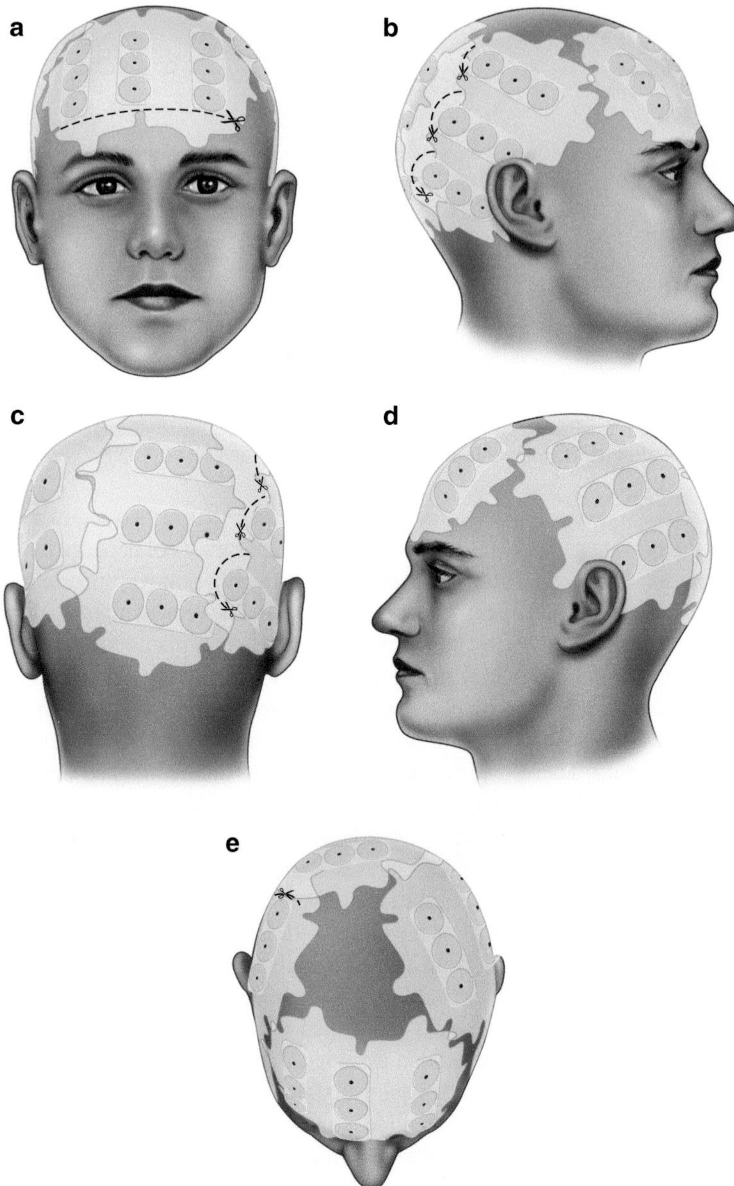


**Fig. 4.3** NovoTAL™ transducer array mapping diagram. Four transducer arrays are arranged orthogonally on the surface of the shaved scalp as seen, from the right-to-left direction, at the (**a**) anterior, (**b**) right, (**c**) posterior, (**d**) left, and (**e**) top configurations

cannot be solved analytically is the Newton-Raphson method [21]. This method is an iterative procedure that minimizes the error each time an approximate solution is computed. Many finite element solvers use an adaptation of the Newton-Raphson method to solve a large number of simultaneous equations by way of organizing them into matrices consisting of many elements. The following is an example of using the Newton-Raphson method to iteratively solve three coupled equations in a $3\times 3$ matrix.

Consider the system of equations written as a vector space of functions:

$$\bar{f}\left(\bar{T}\right)=0, \quad where \;\; \bar{T}=\left(x,y,z\right)\therefore \bar{f}\left(x,y,z\right)=\begin{bmatrix} x^2+2y^2+3z^2-3 \\ 2x^2+5y^2-z-1 \\ x+4y+z-7 \end{bmatrix}$$

with an initial guess $\bar{T}^{(0)}=\left(x^{(0)},y^{(0)},z^{(0)}\right)=\left(1,0,1\right)$.

The Jacobian of $\bar{f}\left(x,y,z\right)$ is

$$J_f\left(x,y,z\right)=\nabla\cdot\bar{f}=\begin{bmatrix} \frac{\partial f_1}{\partial x} & \frac{\partial f_1}{\partial y} & \frac{\partial f_1}{\partial z} \\ \frac{\partial f_2}{\partial x} & \frac{\partial f_2}{\partial y} & \frac{\partial f_2}{\partial z} \\ \frac{\partial f_3}{\partial x} & \frac{\partial f_3}{\partial y} & \frac{\partial f_3}{\partial z} \end{bmatrix}=\begin{bmatrix} 2x & 4y & 6z \\ 4x & 10y & -1 \\ 1 & 4 & 1 \end{bmatrix}.$$

Solving the relationship $J_f\left(x^{(k)},y^{(k)},z^{(k)}\right)\left(\bar{T}^{(k+1)}-\bar{T}^{(k)}\right)=-\bar{T}\left(x^{(k)},y^{(k)},z^{(k)}\right)$, where $k$ is the iteration step, requires setting up the problem of interest and substituting the initial guess $\bar{T}^{(0)}$:

$$\begin{bmatrix} 2x & 4y & 6z \\ 4x & 10y & -1 \\ 1 & 4 & 1 \end{bmatrix}\begin{bmatrix} x^{(k+1)}-x^{(k)} \\ y^{(k+1)}-y^{(k)} \\ z^{(k+1)}-z^{(k)} \end{bmatrix}=-\begin{bmatrix} \left(x^{(k)}\right)^2+2\left(y^{(k)}\right)^2+3\left(z^{(k)}\right)^2-3 \\ 2\left(x^{(k)}\right)^2+5\left(y^{(k)}\right)^2-z^{(k)}-1 \\ x^{(k)}+4y^{(k)}+z^{(k)}-7 \end{bmatrix}$$

$$\begin{bmatrix} 2(1) & 4(0) & 6(1) \\ 4(1) & 10(0) & -1 \\ 1 & 4 & 1 \end{bmatrix}\begin{bmatrix} x^{(0+1)}-1 \\ y^{(0+1)}-0 \\ z^{(0+1)}-1 \end{bmatrix}=-\begin{bmatrix} 1 \\ 0 \\ -5 \end{bmatrix}$$

$$\begin{bmatrix} 2 & 0 & 6 \\ 4 & 0 & -1 \\ 1 & 4 & 1 \end{bmatrix} \begin{bmatrix} x^{(1)}-1 \\ y^{(1)}-0 \\ z^{(1)}-1 \end{bmatrix} = -\begin{bmatrix} 1 \\ 0 \\ -5 \end{bmatrix}$$

$$\begin{bmatrix} 2x+0y+6z \\ 4x+0y-z \\ x+4y+z \end{bmatrix} = \begin{bmatrix} 7 \\ 3 \\ 7 \end{bmatrix}$$

Now, the first iterative solution $\overline{T}^{(1)}\left(x^{(1)}, y^{(1)}, z^{(1)}\right)$ consists of:

$$\begin{bmatrix} 2 & 0 & 6 \\ 4 & 0 & -1 \\ 1 & 4 & 1 \end{bmatrix} \begin{bmatrix} x \\ y \\ z \end{bmatrix} = \begin{bmatrix} 7 \\ 3 \\ 7 \end{bmatrix}.$$

At this point, this is similar to a classic linear algebra problem:

$$A^{-1}AX = A^{-1}B$$

$$A^{-1}A = I, \quad \text{where I is the identity matrix } I = \begin{bmatrix} 1 & 0 & 0 \\ 0 & 1 & 0 \\ 0 & 0 & 1 \end{bmatrix}, \quad \textit{so that } IX = X$$

$$\therefore X = A^{-1}B.$$

In order to determine the inverse of matrix $A$, the following definition is used:

$$A^{-1} = \frac{1}{\det(A)} adj(A)$$

For a matrix $A = \begin{bmatrix} a & b & c \\ d & e & f \\ g & h & i \end{bmatrix}$, $\det(A) = a\begin{bmatrix} e & f \\ h & i \end{bmatrix} - b\begin{bmatrix} d & f \\ g & i \end{bmatrix} + c\begin{bmatrix} d & e \\ g & h \end{bmatrix}$

$$\det\begin{bmatrix} 2 & 0 & 6 \\ 4 & 0 & -1 \\ 1 & 4 & 1 \end{bmatrix} = 2\begin{bmatrix} 0 & -1 \\ 4 & 1 \end{bmatrix} - 0\begin{bmatrix} 4 & -1 \\ 1 & 1 \end{bmatrix} + 6\begin{bmatrix} 4 & 0 \\ 1 & 4 \end{bmatrix}$$

$$\det(A) = 2\left[(0\cdot 1)-(-1\cdot 4)\right] - 0\left[(4\cdot 1)-(1\cdot -1)\right] + 6\left[(4\cdot 4)-(1\cdot 0)\right] = 104$$

Now, $adj\ A = Cofactor\ Matrix^{T}$; *where T indicates the transpose operation.*

$$
\begin{aligned}
Cofactor(A) &= \begin{bmatrix} + & - & + \\ - & + & - \\ + & - & + \end{bmatrix} \begin{bmatrix} A_{11} & A_{12} & A_{13} \\ A_{21} & A_{22} & A_{23} \\ A_{31} & A_{23} & A_{33} \end{bmatrix} \\
&= \begin{bmatrix} + & - & + \\ - & + & - \\ + & - & + \end{bmatrix} \begin{bmatrix} \begin{vmatrix} 0 & -1 \\ 4 & 1 \end{vmatrix} & \begin{vmatrix} 4 & -1 \\ 1 & 1 \end{vmatrix} & \begin{vmatrix} 4 & 0 \\ 1 & 4 \end{vmatrix} \\ \begin{vmatrix} 0 & 6 \\ 4 & 1 \end{vmatrix} & \begin{vmatrix} 2 & 6 \\ 1 & 1 \end{vmatrix} & \begin{vmatrix} 2 & 0 \\ 1 & 4 \end{vmatrix} \\ \begin{vmatrix} 0 & 6 \\ 0 & -1 \end{vmatrix} & \begin{vmatrix} 2 & 6 \\ 4 & -1 \end{vmatrix} & \begin{vmatrix} 2 & 0 \\ 4 & 0 \end{vmatrix} \end{bmatrix} \\
&= \begin{bmatrix} + & - & + \\ - & + & - \\ + & - & + \end{bmatrix} \begin{bmatrix} 4 & 5 & 16 \\ -24 & -4 & 8 \\ 0 & -26 & 0 \end{bmatrix} \\
&= \begin{bmatrix} 4 & -5 & 16 \\ 24 & -4 & -8 \\ 0 & 26 & 0 \end{bmatrix}
\end{aligned}
$$

To find the transpose of this cofactor matrix, we have

$$
\begin{bmatrix} 4 & -5 & 16 \\ 24 & -4 & -8 \\ 0 & 26 & 0 \end{bmatrix}^T = \begin{bmatrix} 4 & 24 & 0 \\ -5 & -4 & 26 \\ 16 & -8 & 0 \end{bmatrix}.
$$

We then compute $A^{-1} = \frac{1}{\det(A)} adj(A)$:

$$
A^{-1} = \frac{1}{104} \begin{bmatrix} 4 & 24 & 0 \\ -5 & -4 & 26 \\ 16 & -8 & 0 \end{bmatrix} = \begin{bmatrix} \frac{4}{104} & \frac{24}{104} & 0 \\ -\frac{5}{104} & -\frac{4}{104} & \frac{26}{104} \\ \frac{16}{104} & -\frac{8}{104} & 0 \end{bmatrix} = \begin{bmatrix} \frac{1}{26} & \frac{3}{13} & 0 \\ -\frac{5}{104} & -\frac{1}{26} & \frac{1}{4} \\ \frac{2}{13} & -\frac{1}{13} & 0 \end{bmatrix}
$$

Finally, returning to the original problem,

$$
X = A^{-1}B = \begin{bmatrix} \frac{1}{26} & \frac{3}{13} & 0 \\ -\frac{5}{104} & -\frac{1}{26} & \frac{1}{4} \\ \frac{2}{13} & -\frac{1}{13} & 0 \end{bmatrix} \begin{bmatrix} 7 \\ 3 \\ 7 \end{bmatrix} = \begin{bmatrix} x = \frac{25}{26} \\ y = \frac{135}{104} \\ z = \frac{11}{13} \end{bmatrix} = \overline{T}^{(1)}\left(x^{(1)}, y^{(1)}, z^{(1)}\right)
$$

In order to find an acceptable solution, we repeat the procedure using $\bar{T}^{(k)}$ as the next "guess" until $\bar{T}^{(k+1)}\left(x^{(k+1)}, y^{(k+1)}, z^{(k+1)}\right)$ converges to the same vector $\bar{T}^{(k)}$, or until a desired error tolerance is met. Proof of this concept may be confirmed by computing more iterations as an exercise.

## Solving for the Electric Field Distribution in the Human Head

Though it may be tempting to think that in complex geometry, FEM is the key to solving most applied mathematical problems involving partial differential equations and boundary conditions, such as Maxwell's equations. However, the accuracy of FEM is limited by a number of factors, including the element size, the input parameters, computer hardware and kernel efficiency that represents smoothing of random fluctuations in the iterative solution. As multiple research groups have attempted to solve for the electric field distribution in the human head using FEM, the preparative technique is relatively standardized and involves the use of MR images of a human head for (1) segmentation of various tissue structures, (2) generation of a 3-dimensional mesh for each segmented volume, and (3) importation of the composite mesh into a finite element solver [22–27]. Likewise, the approach to solving for the electric fields is also relatively standardized. This involves (1) identifying and applying physical parameters to different segmented tissue types, (2) specifying appropriate boundary and initial conditions, and (3) solving for the distribution of electric fields, all of which are dependent on the transducer array layout.

## Transducer Array Layout for the Delivery of Tumor Treating Fields

TTFields are delivered via two pairs of transducer arrays placed orthogonally on the shaved surface of the scalp. They are arranged in an anterior-posterior and right-left orientation (Fig. 4.3). Each array has nine circular ceramic disks with a diameter of 2.0 cm and spaced 0.5 cm apart along the short axis and 0.7 cm apart along the long axis. The surface of each ceramic disk has a thin layer of conductive gel that provides good conductivity [28], while nine disks positioned as a 3 × 3 array are secured on the scalp by a larger piece of insulated adhesive tape measuring 14.5 cm × 10.0 cm [29]. TTFields are generated by a battery-powered alternating current generator, operating at 200 kHz with maximum voltage alternating from +50 to −50 V. This generator can be connected to a power cord that is plugged into a regular electric outlet when patients are stationary in bed or chair. It can also be connected to a portable lithium ion battery pack, both of which can be carried by ambulatory patients in a backpack. This portable system currently weighs 7 lb but newer generation of this device will weigh substantially less. The portable battery pack can be

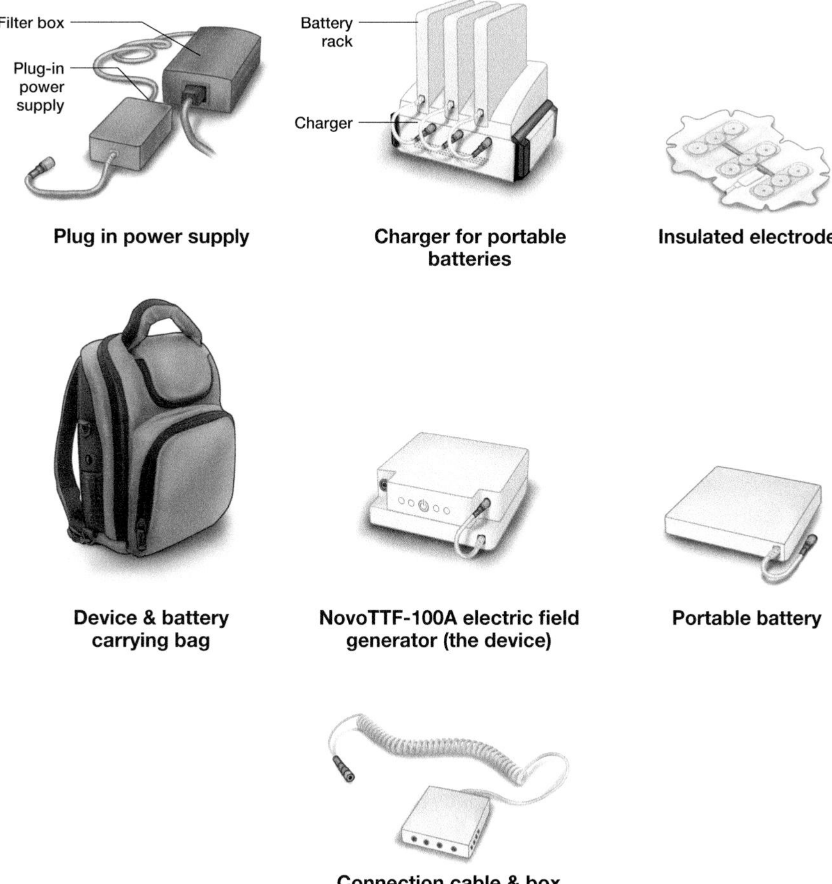


**Fig. 4.4** Overview of the components of the Optune® device as described in the U.S. Food and Drug Administration labeling (http://www.accessdata.fda.gov/cdrh_docs/pdf10/P100034c.pdf)

recharged in a battery charger unit that can simultaneously charge four battery packs and it takes about 6 hours for the battery packs to be fully charged. The components of the Optune® device system are outlined in the U.S. Food and Drug Administration labeling of this device (Fig. 4.4) [29].

The transducer arrays are placed onto patients as shown in Fig. 4.3 according to a placement map generated by proprietary computer software called NovoTAL™ from Novocure. This map is generated based on the head dimensions (anterior-to-posterior, right-to-left, and right-to-midline) and dimensions of a tumor justified to the right border of the head by convention. These measurements submitted into the NovoTAL™ software program allow for the generation of a transducer array placement map. Although the exact method of generating this placement map is not disclosed, it is most likely built on known methods of electrode placement for transcranial direct or alternating current stimulation. Electrode placement for transcranial current stimulation is done by using known conductivity values of the tissues in the head and brain, as well as the conductivity property of the ceramic disk used. Using FEM, the distribution of the electric fields can be estimated by setting the appropriate boundary conditions and material properties, and solving the coupled time-varying Maxwell's equations as explained in Chapter 2 [30]. Various mathematical algorithms such as inverse treatment planning and Monte Carlo simulation can be applied to generate, via an iterative process, the best fit positioning of the arrays [30–32]. Once penetrated into the head, these electric fields are most likely to be distorted by the electric properties of various intracranial structures based on each structure's conductivity and relative permittivity.

## General Procedure for Treatment with Tumor Treating Fields

The U.S. Food and Drug Administration's approval of the Optune® device is currently for patients with recurrent and newly diagnosed glioblastoma. Since the device is self-contained and portable, in practice the patient is undergoing treatment as long as the transducer arrays are continuously in contact with the scalp as directed and powered by the TTFields generator. The positioning of the transducer arrays is currently dictated by NovoTAL™, the array-positioning software provided to the physicians by Novocure, whereas the positioning of the arrays is based on the tumor dimensions as seen on MRI. There is no other treatment planning protocol currently being used for clinical purposes. Once the treating physician or physician assistant reviews the placement procedures and compliance requirements with the patient after informed consent, the arrays are placed onto the scalp and the patient is sent home with the portable battery pack and generator, which are fitted into a small shoulder bag.

## Conclusions

TTFields therapy exerts its anticancer effect by disrupting tumor cell division during metaphase-to-anaphase transition in mitosis. The fields are targeted against α/β tubulin and septin that have large dipole moments, which are necessary for proper cellular division. The visualization of the electric field distribution requires computer modeling that takes into account several intracranial tissue parameters such as spatially varying conductivity and relative permittivity. This is done by segmenting various tissue structures, generating a 3-dimensional mesh for each segmented volume, and importing the composite mesh into a finite element solver, which requires (1) the identification and application of physical parameters to different segmented tissue types, (2) specification of appropriate boundary and initial conditions, and (3) identification of the best solution for the electric field distribution, all of which are dependent on the transducer array layout.

## References


1. Ravant JL, Douki T, Cadet J. Direct and indirect effects of UV radiation on DNA and its components. J Photochem Photobiol B. 2001;63:88–102.
2. Ward JF. DNA damage produced by ionizing radiation in mammalian cells: identities, mechanisms of formation, and reparability. Prog Nucleic Acid Res Mol Biol. 1988;35:95–125.
3. Ward JF. Some biochemical consequences of the spatial distribution of ionizing radiation-produced free radicals. Radiat Res. 1981;86:185–95.
4. Hall E, Giaccia AJ. Radiobiology for the radiologist. 7th ed. Philadelphia: Lippincott Williams & Wilkins; 2012.
5. Riley PA. Free radicals in biology: oxidative stress and the effects of ionizing radiation. Int J Radiat Biol. 1994;65:27–33.
6. Littlefield LG, Kleinerman RA, Sayer AM, Tarone R, Boice Jr JD. Chromosome aberrations in lymphocytes—biomonitors of radiation exposure. Prog Clin Biol Res. 1991;372:387–97.
7. Wong ET, Huberman M, Lu XQ, Mahadevan A. Bevacizumab reverses cerebral radiation necrosis. J Clin Oncol. 2008;26:5649–50.
8. DeAngelis LM, Delattre JY, Posner JB. Radiation-induced dementia in patients cured of brain metastases. Neurology. 1989;39:789–96.
9. Wong CS, Fehlings MG, Sahgal A. Pathobiology of radiation myelopathy and strategies to mitigate injury. Spinal Cord. 2015;53:574–80.
10. Felder CE, Prilusky J, Silman I, Sussman JL. A server and database for dipole moments of proteins. Nucleic Acids Res. 2007;35:512–21.
11. Kirson ED, Gurvich Z, Schneiderman R, et al. Disruption of cancer cell replication by alternating electric fields. Cancer Res. 2004;64:3288–95.
12. Gera N, Yang A, Holtzman TS, et al. Tumor treating fields perturb the localization of septins and cause aberrant mitotic exit. PLoS One. 2015;10:e0125269.
13. Lee SX, Wong ET, Swanson KD. Mitotic interference of cancer cells during anaphase by electric field from NovoTTF-100A. Neuro-Oncology. 2011;13:iii13–4.
14. Lee SX, Wong ET, Swanson KD. Disruption of cell division within anaphase by tumor treating electric fields (TTFields) leads to immunogenic cell death. Neuro Oncol. 2013;15:iii66–7.
15. Lacouture ME, Davis ME, Elzinga G, et al. Characterization and management of dermatologic adverse events with the NovoTTF-100A system, a novel anti-mitotic electric field device for the treatment of recurrent glioblastoma. Semin Oncol. 2014;41 Suppl 4:S1–14.
16. Clough RW. Early history of the finite element method from the view point of a pioneer. Int J Numer Methods Eng. 2004;60:283–7.
17. Argyris JH, Balmer H, Dolsinis JS, et al. Finite element method—the natural approach. Comput Methods Appl Mech Eng. 1979;17/18:1–106.
18. Zienkiewicz OC, Gago JP, Kelly DW. The hierarchical concept in the finite element method. Comput Struct. 1983;16:53–65.
19. Turner MJ, Clough RW, Martin HC, Topp LJ. Stiffness and deflection analysis of complex structures. J Aeronaut Sci. 1956;23:805–23.
20. Guo D, Fridriksson J, Fillmore P, et al. Automated lesion detection on MRI scans using combined unsupervised and supervised methods. BMC Med Imaging. 2015;15:50.
21. Lindstrom MJ, Bates DM. Newton-Raphson and EM algorithms for linear mixed-effects models for repeated-measures data. J Am Stat Assoc. 1988;83:1014–22.
22. Miranda PC, Kekkonen R, Salvador R, et al. Predicting the electric field distribution in the brain for the treatment of glioblastoma. Phys Med Biol. 2014;59:4137–47.

23. Lok E, Hua V, Wong ET. Computed modeling of alternating electric fields therapy for recurrent glioblastoma. Cancer Med. 2015;4:1697–9.
24. Lok E, Swanson KD, Wong ET. Tumor treating fields therapy device for glioblastoma: physics and clinical practice considerations. Expert Rev Med Devices. 2015;12:717–26.
25. Wagner T, Valero-Cabre A, Pascual-Leone A. Noninvasive human brain stimulation. Annu Rev Biomed Eng. 2007;9:527–65.
26. Darvas F, Pantazis D, Kucukaltun-Yildirim E, Leahy RM. Mapping human brain function with MEG and EEG: methods and validation. Neuroimage. 2004;23 Suppl 1:S289–99.
27. Sadleir RJ, Vannorsdall TD, Schretlen DJ, Gordon B. Transcranial direct current stimulation (tDCS) in a realistic head model. Neuroimage. 2010;51:1310–8.
28. McAdams ET, Jossinet J, Lackermeier A, Risacher F. Factors affecting electrode-gel-skin interface impedance in electrical impedance tomography. Med Biol Eng Comput. 1996;34:397–408.
29. Http://Www.Fda.Gov/Ucm/Groups/Fdagov-Public/@Fdagov-Afda-Adcom/Documents/Document/Ucm247168.Pdf.
30. Dmochowski JP, Datta A, Bikson M, Su Y, Parra LC. Optimized multi-electrode stimulation increases focality and intensity at target. J Neural Eng. 2011;8:046011.
31. Datta A, Elwassif M, Battaglia F, Bikson M. Transcranial current stimulation focality using disc and ring electrode configurations: FEM analysis. J Neurol Eng. 2008;5:163–74.
32. Im CH, Jung HH, Choi JD, Lee SY, Jung KY. Determination of optimal electrode positions for transcranial direct current stimulation (tDCS). Phys Med Biol. 2008;53:N219–25.

# Chapter 5
# Response Pattern and Modeling of Tumor Treating Fields

**Josef Vymazal, Aaron M. Rulseh, and Eric T. Wong**

Glioblastoma multiforme (GBM) is the most common primary malignant brain tumor [1, 2], with a global incidence of approximately 3.5 per 100,000 people [2]. Despite standard treatment consisting of surgical resection together with radiotherapy and concomitant/adjuvant temozolomide chemotherapy, the median overall survival (OS) for patients with newly diagnosed GBM is only 12 to 18 months [1–3]. Nearly all patients with GBM experience disease progression despite aggressive first-line therapy, with a median time to progression of 6 to 11 months [1, 4]. Treatment options for GBM at the time of recurrence are limited, and there is no widely accepted standard treatment [4–6]. Thus, new and more effective treatment options are highly desirable.

The Optune® device (Novocure Ltd., Haifa, Israel) is an approved antimitotic treatment for patients with recurrent or newly diagnosed GBM [6–8]. It delivers intermediate-frequency alternating electric fields at 200 kHz, also known as Tumor Treating Fields (TTFields), via noninvasive transducer arrays applied to the scalp based on computerized treatment planning according to anatomic magnetic resonance imaging (MRI) of the tumor [9]. TTFields selectively kill or arrest the

J. Vymazal, M.D., D.Sc. (✉)
Department of Radiology, Na Homolce Hospital, Prague, Czech Republic
e-mail: josef.vymazal@homolka.cz

A.M. Rulseh, M.D., Ph.D.
Department of Radiology, Na Homolce Hospital, Prague, Czech Republic

Department of Radiology, First Medical Faculty, Charles University in Prague, Prague, Czech Republic

E.T. Wong, M.D. (✉)
Division of Neuro-Oncology, Department of Neurology, Beth Israel Deaconess Medical Center, Boston, MA, USA

Department of Physics, University of Massachusetts in Lowell, Lowell, MA 01854, USA
e-mail: ewong@bidmc.harvard.edu



E.T. Wong (ed.), *Alternating Electric Fields Therapy in Oncology*,
DOI 10.1007/978-3-319-30576-9_5

growth of rapidly dividing cells by inhibiting the proper formation of the mitotic spindle and by causing rapid plasma membrane disruption during cytokinesis [10–13]. Therefore, this treatment is selective for dividing cells and requires continuous application for maximal benefit.

## Response Pattern to Tumor Treating Fields

In GBM patients, response is usually characterized by at least a 50 % decrease in the product of the cross-sectional diameter of the tumor [14]. Although response is typically a secondary endpoint in GBM clinical trials, it usually signifies antitumor activity when present. In the initial pilot study of the Optune® device, ten subjects with recurrent GBM were treated with TTFields monotherapy after failing adjuvant temozolomide, while another ten with newly diagnosed GBM received TTFields plus maintenance temozolomide [15]. In the recurrent GBM cohort, there were two *bona fide* responses but their time to response was significantly delayed, with complete response realized in one subject at 6 months and partial response detected in another subject after 14 months [15]. Interestingly, in both tumors initial progression was detected on MRI 1 and 7 months after initiation of TTFields monotherapy. This initial worsening and subsequent shrinkage of the tumor on neuroimaging may be the result of an antitumor immune response as TTFields have been shown to evoke responses in tumor cells that are consistent with immunogenic cell death, including the cell surface expression of calreticulin and secretion of high-mobility group box 1 protein (HMGB1) [16]. Furthermore, TTFields-treated rabbits with implanted VX2 tumors in the sub-renal capsule had a reduced number of metastases to the lungs and these metastases had a significant increase in immune infiltrates [17].

In the phase III trial for recurrent GBM, 237 subjects were randomized in a 1:1 fashion to receive TTFields monotherapy ($n = 120$) or best physician's choice chemotherapy ($n = 117$) [6]. There were 14 responders, 3 complete and 11 partial responses, in the TTFields monotherapy cohort and 6 of them experienced initial tumor growth at an interval of 2 to 24 months while on treatment [6, 18]. The median time to response and the response duration in these patients were longer compared to those who received chemotherapy, 8.4 months versus 5.8 months and 7.3 months versus 5.6 months, respectively [18]. These findings suggest that responders to TTFields may require a longer time to response but, once initiated, they have a more durable response than those treated with chemotherapy. These findings in the phase III trial for recurrent GBM also provide support for an immune-mediated component in the mechanism for TTFields' anti-GBM efficacy.

By combining the participants from both trials for recurrent GBM, there were a total of 16 responders, 2 from the pilot study and 14 from the phase III registration trial [6, 15]. As shown in Fig. 5.1, the median time to objective radiographic response in the 16 responders was 5.2 months (95 % CI 3.2–7.6 months), the median response duration was 12.9 months, and the median overall survival was 26.5 months. Figures 5.2, 5.3, 5.4, and 5.5 show exemplary post-gadolinium-enhanced

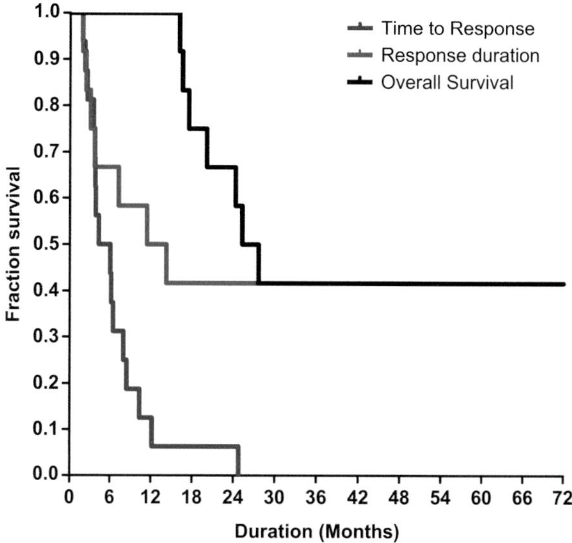


**Fig. 5.1** Kaplan-Meier estimates of the time to radiological response according to Macdonald criteria (*blue*), response duration (*red*), and overall survival (*black*) of the 16 responders combined from the pilot study and the phase III trial for recurrent GBM [6, 15]. Vymazal et al. Response patterns of recurrent glioblastomas treated with tumor-treating fields. Semin Oncol. 41 Suppl 6:S14-S24, 2014. Elsevier

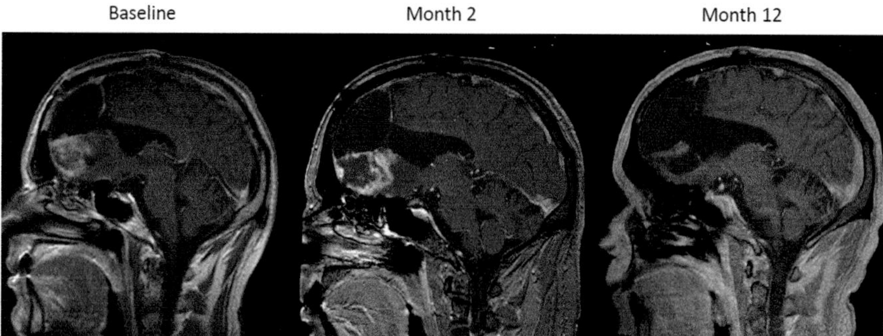


**Fig. 5.2** T1-weighted post-contrast MR images of a 48-year-old man with prior grade II astrocytoma, which transformed to GBM as confirmed by tissue biopsy. The subject progressed after receiving radiotherapy with concomitant temozolomide followed by 3 cycles of adjuvant temozolomide. He subsequently responded to TTFields, achieved at 12 months, and remained stable for an additional 20 months while on treatment. Vymazal et al. Response patterns of recurrent glioblastomas treated with tumor-treating fields. Semin Oncol. 41 Suppl 6:S14-S24, 2014. Elsevier

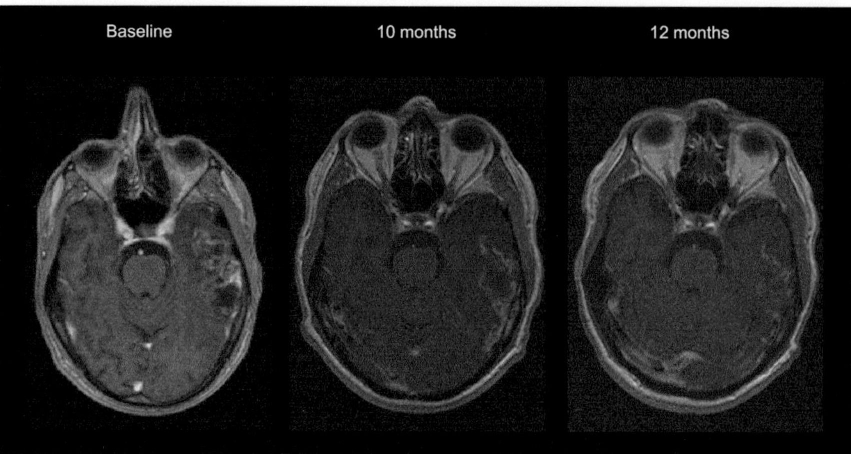


**Fig. 5.3** T1-weighted post-contrast MR images of a 51-year-old man with primary GBM which recurred 6 months after chemoradiotherapy with temozolomide. The patient underwent a biopsy of the tumor only without surgical resection. He had a very gradual response, reaching a 50 % reduction in tumor size after 10 months on TTFields. He remained stable for an additional 2 months on treatment. Vymazal et al. Response patterns of recurrent glioblastomas treated with tumor-treating fields, Semin Oncol. 41 Suppl 6:S14-S24, 2014. Elsevier

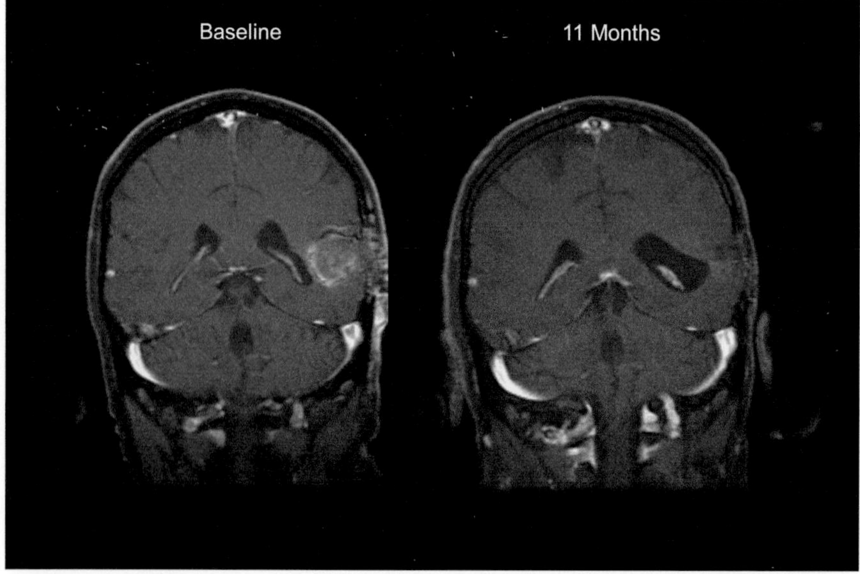


**Fig. 5.4** T1-weighted post-contrast MR images of a 55-year-old man with primary GBM which recurred for the third time after receiving radiotherapy with concomitant temozolomide, 2 cycles of adjuvant temozolomide, 3 cycles of bevacizumab with irinotecan, and 1 cycle of erlotinib and sorafenib. The subject had a partial response after 4 months of treatment with TTFields and remained stable for an additional 8 months while on therapy. Vymazal et al. Response patterns of current glioblastomas treated with tumor-treating fields. Semin Oncol. 41 Suppl 6:S14-S24, 2014. Elsevier

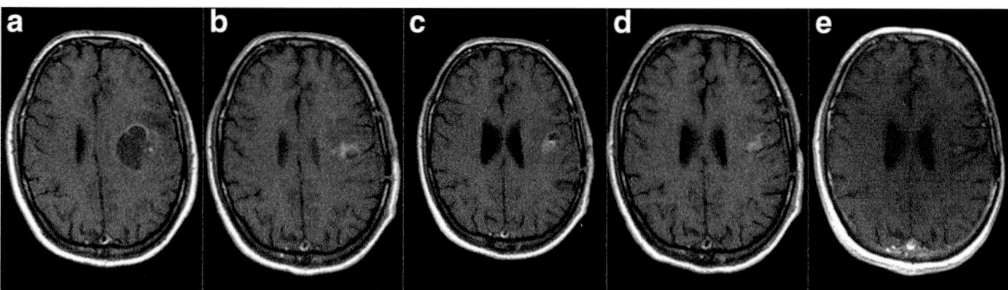


**Fig. 5.5** T1-weighted post-contrast MR images of a 41-year-old man with GBM which recurred following partial surgical resection and radiotherapy with concomitant daily temozolomide. (**a**) Before initial surgery, GBM was detected on MRI in the left frontal region. (**b**) Seven months after initial diagnosis, an enhancing lesion suspected to be recurrent or residual tumor was detected and treatment with the Optune® device was initiated. (**c**) Seven months after initiation of TTFields, the enhancing lesion became partly cystic. (**d**) Ten months after initiation of TTFields, regression of the cystic portion of the lesion was detected, but a subtle enhancement was still present. (**e**) The faintly enhancing region remains without progression 94 months after initiation of TTFields. *GBM* glioblastoma multiforme, *MR* magnetic resonance, *TTFields* Tumor Treating Fields. Rulseh et al. Long-term survival of patients suffering from glioblastoma multiforme treated with tumor-treating fields. World J Surg Oncol. 10:220, 2012. BioMed Central

T1-weighted MR images of responders. The most important findings were that responses to TTField treatment developed relatively slowly and, in most cases, the responses were remarkably durable.

In 7 of the 16 responders (44 %) from both studies, MRI showed initial tumor growth. Exemplary MR images of delayed responders can be found in Figs. 5.6 and 5.7. Median time to reversal of tumor growth in delayed responders was 4 (95 % CI 2.3–7.4) months. Initial tumor growth was accompanied by an increase in T2-weighted signal intensity in 5 of the 7 delayed responders (71 %) (Fig. 5.6). Diffusion-weighted imaging in 3 of the 7 delayed responders did not demonstrate increased signal in the first 4 months after treatment initiation. The averaged maximal tumor area over time compared to baseline in the delayed responders is shown in Fig. 5.8.

There was a correlation between response and prolonged survival in both cohorts in the trial, and responders treated with either TTFields monotherapy or chemotherapy lived longer than nonresponders. In the cohort treated with TTFields, the median overall survival was 24.8 months for responders and 6.2 for nonresponders, while it was 20.0 months for responders and 6.8 months for nonresponders in the cohort received chemotherapy [18]. Of note, a significant Pearson correlation was only found between time to response and overall survival, as well as between response duration and overall survival, in the TTFields cohort but not the chemotherapy cohort [18]. This suggests that a response in the TTFields-treated subjects predicts prolonged survival but this is not necessarily so for chemotherapy-treated subjects. In fact, 3 of the responders to TTFields in the phase III trial lived more than 40 months from the time of recurrence and 2 in pilot trial survived longer than 72 months from the time of treatment initiation [15, 18].

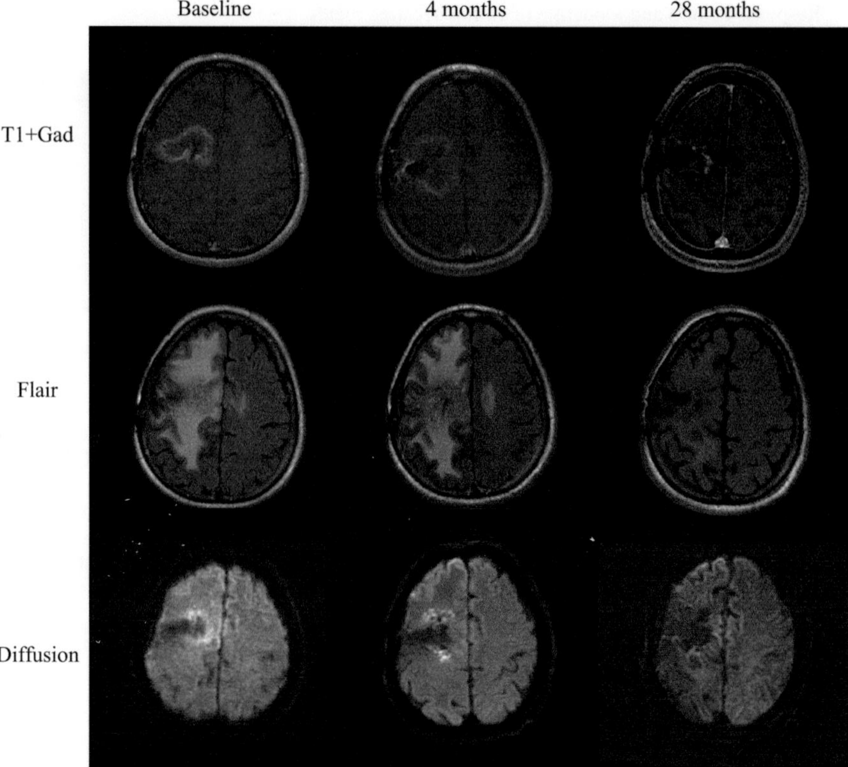


**Fig. 5.6** T1-weighted post-contrast with corresponding FLAIR and diffusion MR images of a heavily pretreated 48-year-old man with secondary GBM. The patient underwent 3 debulking surgeries, radiotherapy with concomitant daily temozolomide, as well as Gamma knife boost. The tumor showed heterozygous deletions of 1p and 19q chromosomes and methylated *MGMT* promoter. The patient was treated with TTFields for 28 months until radiological response was achieved and has been on treatment for 45 months thus far. Notably, the tumor grew during the first 8 months on treatment and only then began to decrease in size. Additional MRI sequences show that the initial tumor growth was accompanied by increased FLAIR signal but not increased diffusion signal. Vymazal et al. Response patterns of recurrent glioblastomas treated with tumor-treating fields. Semin Oncol. 41 Suppl 6:S14-S24, 2014. Elsevier

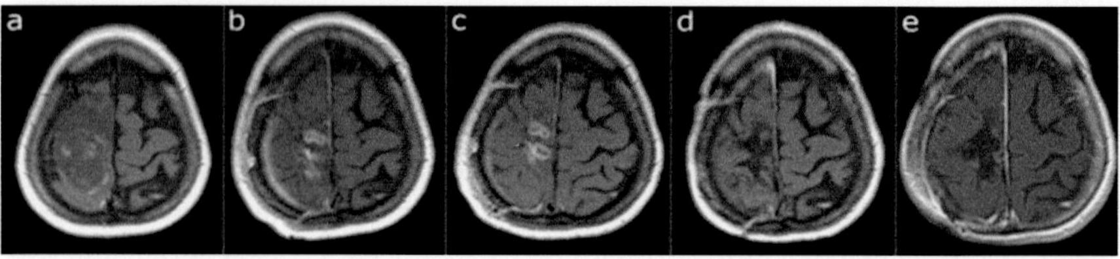


**Fig. 5.7** T1-weighted post-contrast MR images of a 52-year-old woman with GBM, which recurred following surgical resection and radiotherapy with concomitant daily temozolomide. (**a**) GBM was identified in the right central region before initial surgery. (**b**) Three months following surgery and after radiotherapy with concomitant daily temozolomide, two enhancing lesions suspected to be recurrent tumor were detected. (**c**) One month after initiation of TTFields, the caudal enhancing lesion increased in size. (**d**) Six months after initiation of TTFields, both enhancing lesions regressed in size. (**e**) Both lesions underwent complete regression 8 months after initiation of TTFields and have remained so for another 117 months. Rulseh, et al. Long-term survival of patients suffering from glioblastoma multiforme treated with tumor-treating fields. World J Surg Oncol. 10:220, 2012. BioMed Central

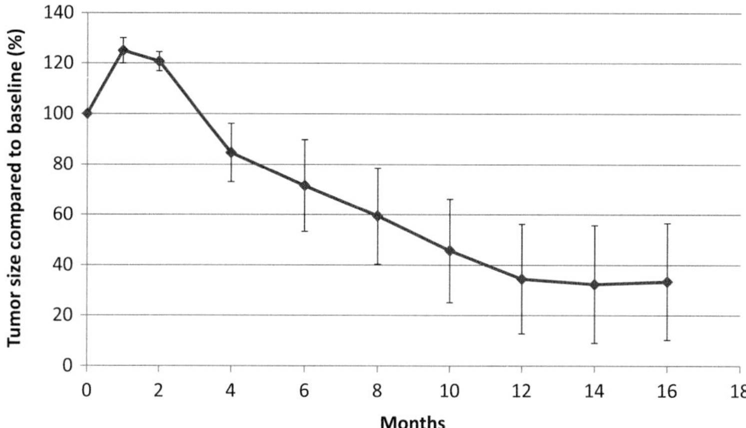


**Fig. 5.8** Time course of normalized tumor size in the 7 delayed responders to TTFields. Data are presented as average tumor area ± standard deviation normalized to baseline, or pretreatment, tumor area. Vymazal et al. Response Patterns of Current Glioblastomas Treated with Tumor-Treating Fields. Semin Oncol. 41:S14-S24. 2014. Elsevier

## Predictive Factors for Response to Tumor Treating Fields

Despite responders to TTFields having similar baseline characteristics to the rest of the population in both trials [15, 18], there may be other factors correlated to radiological response, which continue to be the subject of active investigation. First, an increase in treatment compliance was associated with better response and longer overall survival [19]. This is most likely due to TTFields' mechanism of action, which only disrupts tumor cells during mitosis at the metaphase-to-anaphase transition, and as a result the Optune® device has to be applied continuously in order to exert benefit [12, 13]. Second, it has been suggested that tumor localization, as well as the internal composition of the tumor, may play a role in treatment response [20, 21]. As the ventricles have high water content and water acts as a conductor for electric fields, the mitotic disruption effect of TTFields may be maximized when the tumor is near the ventricular surface. Third, in the randomized phase III trial, patients with prior low-grade glioma histology, or secondary GBM, had a trend for increased median survival compared to those without [18]. This may be a result of slower rate of tumor growth among patients with secondary GBM [22] and therefore they may have more time for TTFields to exert its antitumor effect. Lastly, patients with GBM need dexamethasone to control neurologic symptoms and this corticosteroid in particular can lead to suppression of multiple immune effector systems that may be required for TTFields-induced tumor rejection [23–25]. Specifically, a *post hoc* analysis of dexamethasone dosage taken by participants of the phase III trial using TTFields monotherapy or chemotherapy for recurrent GBM demonstrated that those who took <4.1 mg/day of dexamethasone lived significantly longer than those who received ≥4.1 mg/day [23]. Taken together, there may be multiple pathways to objective tumor response as a result of TTFields treatment, some of which are intrinsic while others are extrinsic to the patient's tumor.

## Multi-Compartmental Model of Tumor Growth and Delayed Response

To better characterize tumor regression induced by TTFields, Vymazal and Wong [19] constructed a multi-compartmental kinetic model based on the states of cells within the tumor microenvironment, specifically between latency and replication as well as their progression to death and clearance. The model assumed that changes in tumor volume, for any given time interval, are determined by the number of cells in four dynamic compartments: (1) tumor cells in a dormant or latent (L) state, (2) cells that have left the dormant state to enter mitosis and replicate (R), (3) cells that have died (D) within the time interval, and (4) cells that have been cleared (C) from the tumor microenvironment (Fig. 5.9a). Dormant or latent (L) cells are in a reversible transition with the dividing or replicating (R) cells, with forward and reverse rate constants of $k_1$ and $k_2$, respectively. The rate constants are balanced to keep the constituents of the two compartments at a fixed ratio consistent with the histologically determined fraction of dividing cells in GBM tumors. Tumor cells are assumed to die or move to the third compartment through two mechanisms. The first is apoptosis, which mainly depends on nutrient and oxygen supply (blood flow); to simplify the model, a single death rate constant, $k_4$, was used. The second mechanism is the rate of replicating (R) cells progressing to death (D) due to TTFields, which is represented by the rate constant $k_3$. The dead cells are removed from the vascularized layer of the tumor (at least in part via phagocytosis) by transferring them to a virtual fourth compartment with a rate constant $k_5$ (Fig. 5.9a). This model predicted, in GBM tumors continuously exposed to TTFields, a doubling of the baseline tumor volume at 4 weeks before a reduction in tumor volume near 7 months (Fig. 5.9b). This prediction is consistent with the observed tumor behavior, in which there was an initial increase in tumor size that constituted progressive disease, with tumor regression that qualifies as partial response occurring more than 8 months after the initiation of TTFields (Fig. 5.8). Therefore, we may expect that GBM tumors will cease to grow and start to regress in size only after several weeks of continuous exposure. However, objective tumor response may not occur until at least 5 to 8 months later.

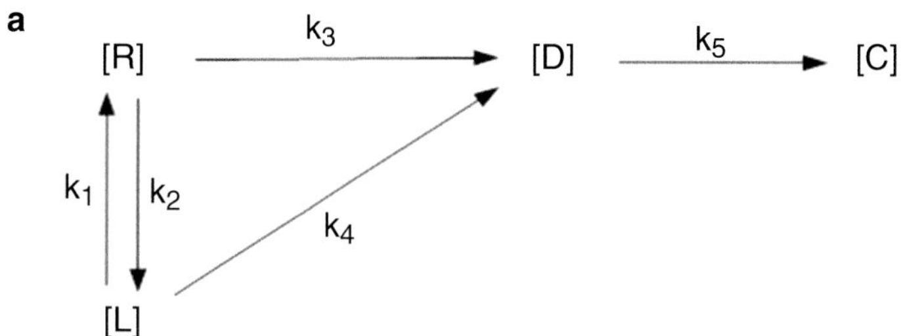


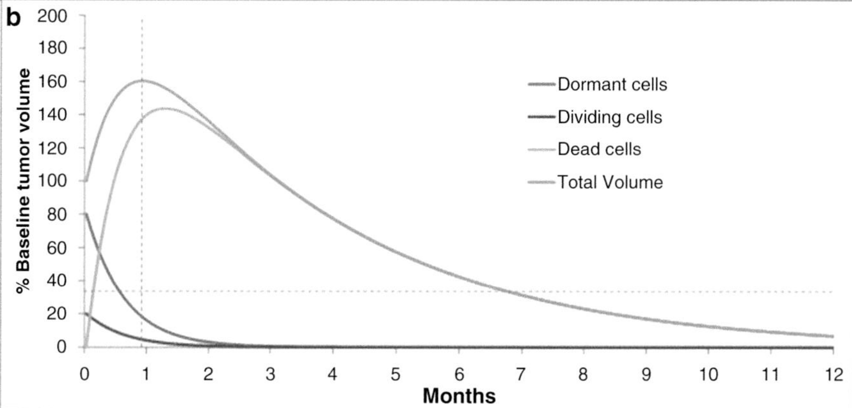


**Fig. 5.9** Multi-compartmental kinetic model of tumor cells. (**a**) Schematic representation of the different compartments in the model and the rate constants associated with the interactions between them. TTFields were modeled as effecting *k3*. [L]=Latent/non-dividing cells; [R]=replicating/dividing cells; [D]=dead cells; [C]=cells cleared from tumor by physiological mechanisms. (**b**) Results of kinetic model simulation and relative changes in tumor compartment size. Volume changes during the initial 9 months of treatment with TTFields are characterized by growth of tumor volume in the initial month, with a maximum near 1 month followed by a gradual decline. A reduction of tumor volume to 35 % is observed at about 6.8 months, equivalent to a 50 % decrease in bi-dimensional tumor measurement or partial response according to the Macdonald or RANO criteria. Dormant cells (*black*); dividing cells (*red*); dead cells (*green*); total tumor volume (*blue*); *vertical dashed line* represents peak tumor volume and time of tumor growth reversal (28 days). Vymazal et al. Response patterns of recurrent glioblastomas treated with tumor-treating fields. Semin Oncol. 41 Suppl 6:S14-S24, 2014. Elsevier

## Conclusion

In summary, TTFields represent a novel treatment option for patients with GBM. Among the trial participants with recurrent GBM, approximately 16 experienced a complete or partial radiological response that typically developed slowly, with a median time to response of 5.2 months, and was generally durable with a median duration of 12.9 months. Some of the responders have lived for 10 years or longer.

Seven of 16 (44 %) GBM responders to TTFields exhibited radiological signs of tumor growth initially, before reversing and regressing in size after a median of 4 months, and a range of 2 to 7 months, of continuous treatment. Therefore, TTFields produce responses slowly and when tumor shrinkage occurs it is often durable. Furthermore, tumor response develops gradually and tumor growth may be observed initially even in eventual responders to this therapy. Thus, we recommend that TTFields should be continued for a sufficient amount of time and that initial radiologic progression following treatment initiation should not be considered a reason to discontinue treatment.

## References


1. Chen J, Xu T. Recent therapeutic advances and insights of recurrent glioblastoma multiforme. Front Biosci (Landmark Ed). 2013;18:676–84.
2. Ostrom QT, Gittleman H, Farah P, Ondracek A, Chen Y, Wolinsky Y, et al. CBTRUS statistical report: primary brain and central nervous system tumors diagnosed in the United States in 2006-2010. Neuro-Oncol. 2013;15 Suppl 2:ii1–56.
3. Cloughesy TF, Cavenee WK, Mischel PS. Glioblastoma: from molecular pathology to targeted treatment. Annu Rev Pathol. 2014;9:1–25.
4. Omuro A, DeAngelis LM. Glioblastoma and other malignant gliomas: a clinical review. JAMA. 2013;310(17):1842–50.
5. Anton K, Baehring JM, Mayer T. Glioblastoma multiforme: overview of current treatment and future perspectives. Hematol Oncol Clin North Am. 2012;26(4):825–53.
6. Stupp R, Wong ET, Kanner AA, et al. NovoTTF-100A versus physician's choice chemotherapy in recurrent glioblastoma: a randomized phase III trial of a novel treatment modality. Eur J Cancer. 2012;48:2192–202.
7. Fonkem E, Wong ET. NovoTTF-100A: a new treatment modality for recurrent glioblastoma. Expert Rev Neurother. 2012;12(8):895–9.
8. Stupp R, Tallibert S, Kanner AA, et al. Maintenance therapy with tumor-treating fields plus temozolomide vs temozolomide alone for glioblastoma: a randomized clinical trial. JAMA. 2015;314:2535–43.
9. Http://Www.Fda.Gov/Ucm/Groups/Fdagov-Public/@Fdagov-Afda-Adcom/Documents/Document/Ucm247168.Pdf.
10. Davies AM, Weinberg U, Palti Y. Tumor treating fields: a new frontier in cancer therapy. Ann N Y Acad Sci. 2013;1291:86–95.
11. Kirson ED, Dbaly V, Tovarys F, Vymazal J, Soustiel JF, Itzhaki A, et al. Alternating electric fields arrest cell proliferation in animal tumor models and human brain tumors. Proc Natl Acad Sci U S A. 2007;104(24):10152–7.
12. Kirson ED, Gurvich Z, Schneiderman R, Dekel E, Itzhaki A, Wasserman Y, et al. Disruption of cancer cell replication by alternating electric fields. Cancer Res. 2004;64(9):3288–95.
13. Gera N, Yang A, Holtzman TS, et al. Tumor treating fields perturb the localization of septins and cause aberrant mitotic exit. PLoS One. 2015;10:e0125269.
14. Hess KR, Wong ET, Jaeckle KA, et al. Response and progression in recurrent malignant glioma. Neuro-Oncology. 1999;1:282–8.
15. Rulseh AM, Keller J, Klener J, Sroubek J, Dbaly V, Syrucek M, et al. Long-term survival of patients suffering from glioblastoma multiforme treated with tumor treating fields. World J Surg Oncol. 2012;10(1):220.

16. Lee SX, Wong ET, Swanson KD. Disruption of cell division within anaphase by tumor treating electric fields (TTFields) leads to immunogenic cell death. Neuro-Oncology. 2013;15:iii66–7.
17. Kirson ED, Giladi M, Gurvich Z, et al. Alternating electric fields (TTFields) inhibit metastatic spread of solid tumors to the lungs. Clin Exp Metastasis. 2009;26:633–40.
18. Wong ET, Lok E, Swanson KD, et al. Response assessment of NovoTTF-100A versus best physician's choice chemotherapy in recurrent glioblastoma. Cancer Med. 2014;3:592–602.
19. Vymazal J, Wong ET. Response patterns of recurrent glioblastomas treated with tumor-treating fields. Semin Oncol. 2014;41 Suppl 6:S14–24.
20. Miranda PC, Mekonnen A, Salvador R, Basser PJ. Predicting the electric field distribution in the brain for the treatment of glioblastoma. Phys Med Biol. 2014;59:4137–47.
21. Lok E, Hua V, Wong ET. Computed modeling of alternating electric fields therapy for recurrent glioblastoma. Cancer Med. 2015;4:1697–9.
22. Ohgaki H, Dessen P, Jourde B, et al. Genetic pathways to glioblastoma: a population-based study. Cancer Res. 2004;64:6892–9.
23. Wong ET, Lok E, Gautam S, Swanson KD. Dexamethasone exerts profound immunologic interference on treatment efficacy for glioblastoma. Br J Cancer. 2015;113:232–41.
24. Benedetti S, Pirola B, Poliani PL, et al. Dexamethasone inhibits the anti-tumor effect of interleukin 4 on rat experimental gliomas. Gene Ther. 2003;10:188–92.
25. Fauci AS. Mechanisms of corticosteroid action on lymphocyte subpopulation. II. Differential effects of in vivo hydrocortisone, prednisone and dexamethasone on the in vitro expression of lymphocyte function. Clin Exp Immunol. 1976;24:54–62.

# Chapter 6
# Clinical Efficacy of Tumor Treating Fields for Recurrent Glioblastoma

**Eric T. Wong**

Recurrent glioblastoma is typically identified based on an increase in size or presence of new tumor as seen on neuroimaging. In recurrent primary glioblastoma [1], the pathology is already established at initial diagnosis and, therefore, a neurosurgical procedure for the purpose of obtaining additional tissue solely for diagnosis is not necessary. However, in secondary glioblastoma, tissue confirmation is indicated when the prior diagnosis is a low-grade or anaplastic glioma [2]. If the patient previously had radiotherapy, confirming a glioblastoma diagnosis can be challenging because radiation-induced necrosis or hyalinized vasculature is not enough, while tumor-associated pseudopalisading necrosis or multicellular vascular hyperplasia is absolutely needed. Additionally, a definition of tumor growth has been established by the Macdonald criteria [3] and, more recently, by the Response Assessment in Neuro-Oncology (RANO) criteria [4]. Both use 2-dimensional measurement as defined by the product of the largest perpendicular diameters of the tumor on MRI. Although Macdonald criteria define enhancement on post-gadolinium T1-weighted image as the region of tumor, RANO differs in the definition of tumor by including provisions to account for a lack of enhancement when patients are on antiangiogenesis therapies [5] or, in cases of pseudoprogression, too much enhancement that occurs after radiation and concomitant temozolomide [6]. Despite these generally accepted criteria, invasion by microscopic tumor cells into the adjacent brain that cannot be readily detected on MRI is a major hallmark of progressing glioblastoma [7].

Survival is limited at the time of recurrence in glioblastoma patients and their ability to maintain tumor stability from treatment is compromised. Median overall survival (OS) is a dismal 25 weeks and median progression-free survival (PFS) is only 9 weeks [8]. A majority of patients are debilitated to such an extent that no

E.T. Wong, M.D. (✉)
Division of Neuro-Oncology, Department of Neurology, Beth Israel Deaconess Medical Center, Boston, MA, USA

Department of Physics, University of Massachusetts in Lowell, Lowell, MA 01854, USA
e-mail: ewong@bidmc.harvard.edu



E.T. Wong (ed.), *Alternating Electric Fields Therapy in Oncology*,
DOI 10.1007/978-3-319-30576-9_6

further treatment would benefit them. For those who have preserved neurologic functions, typically defined as a Karnofsky performance status of 70 or better, aggressive treatments may preserve their neurological functions. Surgery's role is limited unless 90 % or more of the tumor can be removed safely to achieve a survival benefit [9], while carmustine-impregnated dissolvable polymer wafers, which are implanted into the cavity of the resected tumor, are the only intervention for recurrent glioblastoma that showed a slight survival advantage in a randomized phase III trial [10]. Radiosurgery can be performed on tumors that are small and well circumscribed, but this intervention is not believed to lengthen patient survival [11, 12]. Bevacizumab, a monoclonal antibody against vascular endothelial growth factor, is the most commonly used drug in this population [5]. Although it has a high radiographic response rate and can provide a period of neurologic stabilization and even improvement, bevacizumab also does not appear to make patients live longer [13, 14]. Therefore, new treatments are needed.

Tumor Treating Fields (TTFields) are another modality of anticancer treatment that use alternating electric fields at 200 kHz to disrupt tumor cell cytokinesis as they progress from metaphase to anaphase during mitosis [15, 16]. There are a number of downstream consequences, including (1) violent blebbing of the cytoplasmic membrane, (2) asymmetric chromosome segregation, (3) endoplasmic reticulum stress that leads to the upregulation of chaperonin such as calreticulin on the surface of cells, (4) immune recognition of disrupted cells, and (5) eventual immunogenic cell death mediated by either the innate or the adaptive immune system [16, 17]. The key proteins that trigger all these downstream effects are thought to be critical for mitosis, and they perform functions specific at the space and time domains near the end of metaphase and the beginning of anaphase. Furthermore, in order for such proteins to be influenced by TTFields at 200 kHz, they must possess a large dipole moment such that their disrupted functions will result in mitotic failure. Two such proteins, septin and tubulin, fit this profile and they have dipole moments of 2711 and 1660 Debyes [18]. Septin is a large heterotrimeric protein complex that helps organize the cytokinetic cleavage furrow in anaphase [19], while tubulin mediates the segregation of sister chromatids to the opposing centrioles [20]. Septin appears to have a stronger influence on this process because of its larger dipole moment and its disruption triggers violent cytoplasmic blebbing that may precede the segregation of sister chromatids. Furthermore, it is the mode of cell death mediated by the immune system, which is a consequence of the induction of cytoplasmic stress and the translocation of endoplasmic chaperonin to the tumor cell surface facilitating immune recognition, that is the critical process translatable into clinical efficacy [17].

## Pilot Study of Tumor Treating Fields in Recurrent Glioblastoma

The first-in-human trial was a pilot study, conducted from 2004 to 2005, to evaluate the safety and efficacy of TTFields therapy in 10 patients with recurrent glioblastoma [21]. The most common adverse event was contact dermatitis that occurred in the majority and was caused by hydrogel-induced irritation of the scalp. Two patients experienced tumor-related partial seizures. No hematologic or electrolyte toxicity was seen, except for elevated liver enzymes in those taking anticonvulsants. The median overall survival of the 10 patients was 14.4 months and the 1-year survival rate was 67.5 % [21]. The median time to tumor progression was 6.0 months [21]. There was one complete and one partial responder who were still alive, respectively, at 84 and 87 months from treatment initiation [22]. Furthermore, the intensity of electric fields as directly measured in another patient was validated to be within 10 % of the values estimated by computer modeling, suggesting that TTFields applied on the scalp were able to penetrate into the intracranial compartments [21].

## EF-11 was the First Randomized Trial Utilizing Tumor Treating Fields

The EF-11 phase III trial was conducted between 2006 and 2009 comparing TTFields monotherapy versus Best Physician's Choice chemotherapy. The primary endpoint was OS and secondary endpoints included PFS, response rate, and quality of life assessment [23]. In the intent-to-treat population, the median OS was 6.6 months for TTFields compared to 6.0 months for chemotherapy, with a hazard ratio of 0.86 ($p=0.27$) (Fig. 6.1). About 31 % of the chemotherapy cohort received bevacizumab alone or in combination with chemotherapy. The median PFS of TTFields and chemotherapy was 2.2 months and 2.1 months, respectively, with a hazard ratio

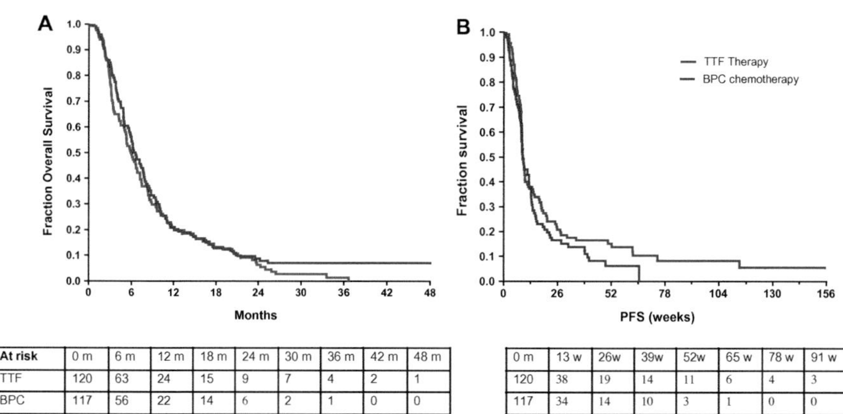


| At risk | 0 m | 6 m | 12 m | 18 m | 24 m | 30 m | 36 m | 42 m | 48 m |
|---|---|---|---|---|---|---|---|---|---|
| TTF | 120 | 63 | 24 | 15 | 9 | 7 | 4 | 2 | 1 |
| BPC | 117 | 56 | 22 | 14 | 6 | 2 | 1 | 0 | 0 |

| 0 m | 13 w | 26w | 39w | 52w | 65 w | 78 w | 91 w |
|---|---|---|---|---|---|---|---|
| 120 | 38 | 19 | 14 | 11 | 6 | 4 | 3 |
| 117 | 34 | 14 | 10 | 3 | 1 | 0 | 0 |

**Fig. 6.1** Survival outcome in subjects enrolled in the EF-11 trial. Kaplan-Meier estimates of overall survival (**A**) and progression-free survival (**B**) in the TTFields monotherapy and Best Physician's Choice chemotherapy cohorts in the EF-11 phase III trial. From Stupp et al. NovoTTF-100A versus physician's choice chemotherapy in recurrent glioblastoma: A randomised phase III trial of a novel treatment modality. Eur J Cancer 48: 2192-2202, 2012. With permission from Elsevier

of 0.81 ($p = 0.16$). In addition, the results demonstrated that the PFS at 6 months was 21.4 and 15.1 %, respectively ($p = 0.13$). One-year survival rate was 20 % in both cohorts. The outcome of the trial indicates that TTFields have comparable efficacy when compared to chemotherapy and bevacizumab.

The most common adverse events associated with the device were grade 1 or 2 scalp irritation. Shifting of the arrays slightly during array change and applying topical corticosteroid can minimize this side effect [24]. There were far less hematological toxicities; other reported adverse events included appetite loss, constipation, diarrhea, fatigue, nausea, vomiting, and pain, which were associated with chemotherapy. Furthermore, additional analyses showed that device-treated patients had better cognitive and emotional functions. Based on the comparable efficacy results, superior safety profile, and a better quality of life, the U.S. Food and Drug Administration approved the Optune® device on April 8, 2011 for the treatment of recurrent glioblastoma.

## *Post Hoc* Analysis of Prognostic Factors

The apparent discrepancy in the OS rates between the pilot study and the phase III trial prompted a series of *post hoc* analyses of the trial data. The first analysis centered on responders and it revealed two important characteristics. First, 5 of 14 responders treated with TTFields monotherapy had prior low-grade histology while none of the 7 responders treated with chemotherapy had that [25]. Second, the analysis revealed significantly less dexamethasone use in responders compared to nonresponders [25]. Responders in the TTFields monotherapy group received a median dexamethasone dose of 1.0 mg/day compared to nonresponders who received 5.2 mg/day ($p = 0.0019$). Similar differences were also noted in the median cumulative dexamethasone dose of 7.1 mg for responders versus 261.7 mg for nonresponders ($p = 0.0041$) (Fig. 6.2). In the chemotherapy cohort, the median dexamethasone dose used was 1.2 mg/day for responders versus 6.0 mg/day for nonresponders ($p < 0.0001$). However, the median cumulative dexamethasone dose was not significantly different, 348.5 mg for responders versus 242.3 mg for nonresponders ($p = 0.9520$) (Fig. 6.3). These data suggest that TTFields efficacy may be influenced by concurrent dexamethasone use, which is a clinically modifiable factor in the patient. This finding prompted an in-depth analysis of the dexamethasone effect in the entire trial population.

An unsupervised modified binary search algorithm was used to stratify the TTFields monotherapy arm of EF-11 based on the dexamethasone dosage that provided the greatest statistical difference in survival (Fig. 6.3). This analysis revealed that subjects who used >4.1 mg/day of dexamethasone had a markedly shortened median OS of 4.8 months as compared to those received ≤4.1 mg/day, who had a median OS of 11.0 months ($\chi^2 = 34.6$, $p < 0.0001$) [26]. Subjects in the chemotherapy arm were observed to have a similar, but less robust, dichotomization and those who used >4.1 and ≤4.1 mg/day of dexamethasone had respective median OS of 6.0 and 8.9 months ($\chi^2 = 10.0$, $p = 0.0015$). This difference in OS based on dexamethasone dose was unrelated to tumor size and most likely due to dexamethasone's interference with patient immune effector functions (Fig. 6.4). This notion was supported by

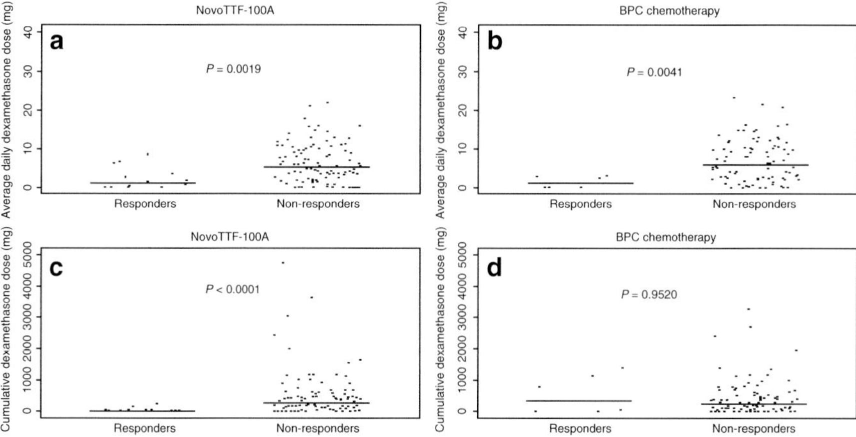


**Fig. 6.2** Scatterplot of mean daily dexamethasone and cumulative dexamethasone dose in responders and nonresponders. (**a**) In the TTFields monotherapy cohort, the respective median and mean daily dexamethasone dose was 1.0 and 2.3 (95 % CI 0.8–3.8) mg for responders versus 5.2 and 6.8 (95 % CI 5.6–8.1) mg for nonresponders ($p=0.0019$). (**b**) In the BPC chemotherapy cohort, the respective median and mean daily dexamethasone dose was 1.2 and 1.4 (95 % CI 0.3–2.4) mg for responders versus 6.0 and 7.2 (95 % CI 6.0–8.4) mg for nonresponders ($p=0.0041$). (c) In the TTFields monotherapy cohort, the respective median and mean cumulative dexamethasone dose was 7.1 and 35.9 (95 % CI N/A to 72.5) mg for responders versus 261.7 and 485.6 (95 % CI 347.9–623.4) mg for nonresponders ($p<0.0001$). (**d**) In the BPC chemotherapy cohort, the respective median and mean cumulative dexamethasone dose was 348.5 and 525.6 (95 % CI 96.5–954.7) mg for responders versus 242.3 and 431.0 (95 % CI 328.1–533.8) mg for nonresponders ($p=0.9520$). *BPC* Best Physician's Choice, *CI* confidence interval, *N/A* not available, *TTFields* Tumor Treating Fields. Wong et al. Response Assessment of versus best physician's choice chemotherapy in recurrent glioblastoma. Cancer Med. 3(3): 592-602, 2014. John Wiley and Sons

a single-institution validation cohort of patients treated with TTFields, using their $CD3^+$, $CD4^+$, and $CD8^+$ T lymphocytes as a marker of immune competency, and that showed their survival was impaired by a lower lymphocyte count suggesting immune competency is an important factor for TTFields efficacy (Fig. 6.4). In addition, a dexamethasone dosage of >4.0 mg/day, used by patients who were undergoing concomitant radiotherapy and daily temozolomide for their newly diagnosed glioblastoma, was also found to be a poor prognostic factor further supporting the conclusion that dexamethasone can impair the efficacy of treatment used in this population [27]. In both cohorts of the EF-11 trial, successive increases in dexamethasone usage above 4.1 mg/day were associated with progressive decrements in survival up to an inflection point near 8.0 mg/day, after which the rate of survival decreased slowly thereafter. Taken together, these data indicate that dexamethasone exerts a generalized and profound interference on the efficacy of both TTFields and chemotherapies against glioblastoma. Therefore, dexamethasone use should be aggressively minimized and other groups have since substantiated our finding [28, 29].

A re-analysis of the intent-to-treat population in EF-11 was performed to account for the insufficient treatment effect in 27 subjects who received less than 1 month or less than 1 cycle of TTFields monotherapy. This is because the antitumor effect of TTFields requires continuous administration, while chemotherapy can exert its effi-

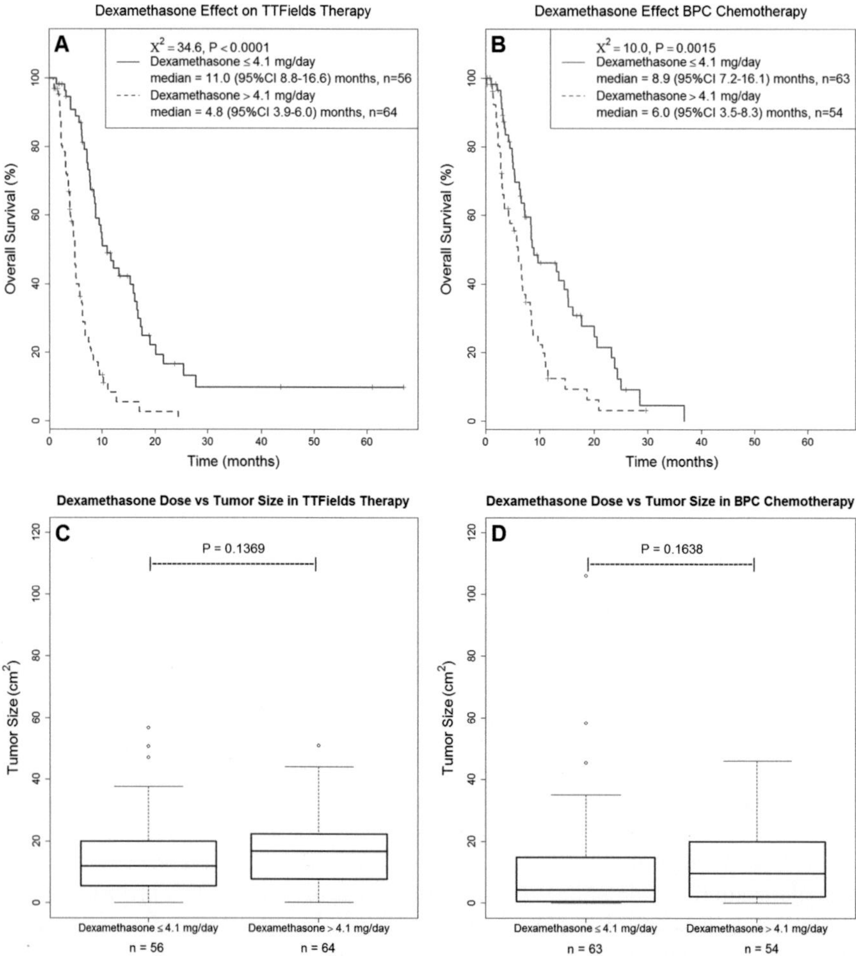


**Fig. 6.3** Survival outcome stratified by dexamethasone dosage. Kaplan-Meier OS and tumor size with respect to dexamethasone requirement of ≤4.1 mg/day versus >4.1 mg/day from subjects enrolled in the phase III trial comparing TTFields versus BPC chemotherapy. (**A**) Subjects enrolled in the TTFields treatment arm taking dexamethasone ≤4.1 (*solid blue*) mg/day versus >4.1 (*dashed blue*) mg/day, which was determined by an unsupervised binary partitioning algorithm. Subjects who used ≤4.1 mg/day of dexamethasone ($n$=56) had a median OS of 11.0 months (95 % CI: 8.8–16.6) as compared with those who used >4.1 mg/day ($n$=64) with a median OS of 4.8 months (95 % CI: 3.9–6.0) ($\chi^2$=34.6, $p$<0.0001). (**B**) Subjects enrolled in the BPC chemotherapy arm taking dexamethasone ≤4.1 (*solid red*) mg/day versus >4.1 (*dashed red*) mg/day was determined by the same unsupervised binary partitioning algorithm. Subjects who used ≤4.1 mg/day of dexamethasone ($n$=63) had a median OS of 8.9 months (95 % CI 7.2–16.1) as compared with those who used >4.1 mg/day ($n$=54) with a median OS of 6.0 months (95 % CI 3.5–8.3) ($\chi^2$=10.0, $p$=0.0015). (**C**) Box-and-whisker plot of the bi-dimensional tumor size in the TTFields monotherapy cohort that received dexamethasone ≤4.1 mg/day versus >4.1 mg/day. Subjects who took dexamethasone ≤4.1 mg/day ($n$=56) had a median tumor size of 11.9 (range 0.0–56.7) $cm^2$ as compared with those who used >4.1 mg/day ($n$=64) with a median tumor size of 16.8 (range 0.3–51.0) $cm^2$ ($p$=0.1369). (**D**) Box-and-whisker plot of the bi-dimensional tumor size in the BPC

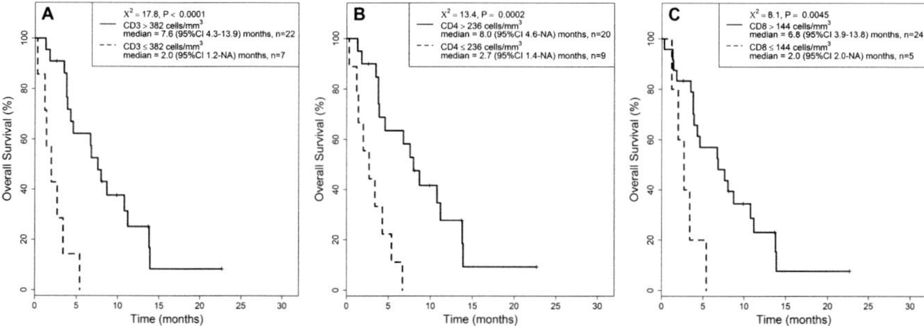


**Fig. 6.4** Kaplan-Meier OS according to the optimal cutoff T-lymphocyte subsets as determined by an unsupervised binary partitioning algorithm. Confirmatory Wilcoxon's rank-sum test was also performed for (**A**) Median OS of patients with absolute CD3⁺ ≤382 cells/mm³ versus >382 cells/mm³ was 2.0 months (range 0.3–5.4) ($n=7$) and 7.7 months (range 1.3–22.7) ($n=25$), respectively ($p=0.0017$). (**B**) Median OS of patients with absolute CD4⁺ ≤236 cells/mm³ versus >236 cells/mm³ was 2.7 months (range 0.3–6.7) ($n=9$) and 8.0 months (range 1.3–22.7) ($n=23$), respectively ($p=0.0029$). (**C**) Median OS of patients with absolute CD8⁺ ≤144 cells/mm³ versus >144 cells/mm³ was 2.7 months (range 1.2–5.4) ($n=5$) and 7.6 months (range 0.3–22.7) ($n=27$), respectively ($p=0.0313$). Data within the graphs were derived from Kaplan-Meier log-rank statistics and showed comparable results when compared to those from Wilconox's rank-sum test. *OS* overall survival. Wong et al. Dexamethasone exerts profound immunologic interference on treatment efficacy for recurrent glioblastoma. Br J Cancer. 113, 232–241, 2015

cacy after administration of just one dose. To make efficacy comparison between the two cohorts in EF-11 more biologically valid, the 27 suboptimally treated subjects were removed and the modified intent-to-treat cohorts consisted of 93 subjects treated with TTFields monotherapy and 117 subjects with chemotherapy [30]. Indeed, the modified TTFields monotherapy arm had a superior overall survival when compared to the chemotherapy arm, median 7.8 months versus 6.0 months, respectively, with a hazard ratio of 0.69 (95 % CI 0.52–0.92) ($p=0.0093$, Fig. 6.5) [30].

Subgroup analyses were also performed in the EF-11 cohort to explore prognostic or predictive factors that may influence survival. First, TTFields treatment compliance significantly correlated with survival. The median overall survival was 5.8, 6.0, and 7.7 months for compliance rate of 40–59 % ($n=10$), 60–79 % ($n=22$), and 80–100 % ($n=77$) ($p=0.039$) (Fig. 6.6) [30]. Second, in the intent-to-treat population, TTFields monotherapy was superior to chemotherapy among the subgroups with prior bevacizumab failure, low-grade glioma, tumor size ≥18 cm², and Karnofsky performance status ≥80 [30]. Lastly, subjects who received TTFields monotherapy ($n=120$) had longer survival compared to those who received bevacizumab-containing regimen ($n=33$), median overall survival 6.6 months versus 4.9 months, respec-

chemotherapy cohort that received dexamethasone ≤4.1 mg/day versus >4.1 mg/day. Subjects who took dexamethasone ≤4.1 mg/day ($n=63$) had a median tumor size of 4.2 (range 0.0–11.2) cm² as compared with those who used >4.1 mg/day ($n=54$) with a median tumor size of 9.6 (range 0.0–46.0) cm² ($p=0.1638$). *BPC* Best Physician's Choice, *OS* overall survival, *TTFields* Tumor Treating Fields, $\chi^2$ chi-square. Wong et al. Dexamethasone exerts profound immunologic interference on treatment efficacy for recurrent glioblastoma. Br J Cancer. 113, 232-241, 2015.

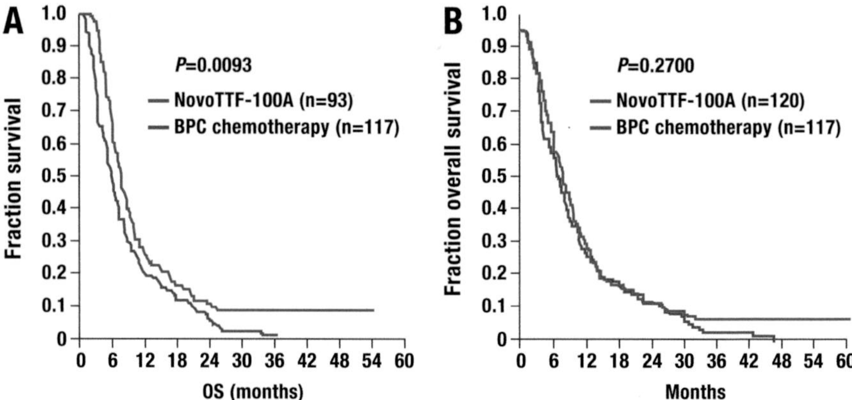


**Fig. 6.5** Kaplan-Meier overall survival for (**A**) mITT and (**B**) ITT populations with recurrent glioblastoma treated with TTFields monotherapy or BPC chemotherapy in the EF-11 phase III trial. *BPC* best physician's choice, *ITT* intent to treat, *mITT* modified intent to treat. From Kanner et al. *Post Hoc* analyses of intention-to-treat population in phase III comparison of NovoTTF-100A™ system versus best physician's choice chemotherapy. Semin Oncol. 41:S25-S34, 2014. With permission from Elsevier

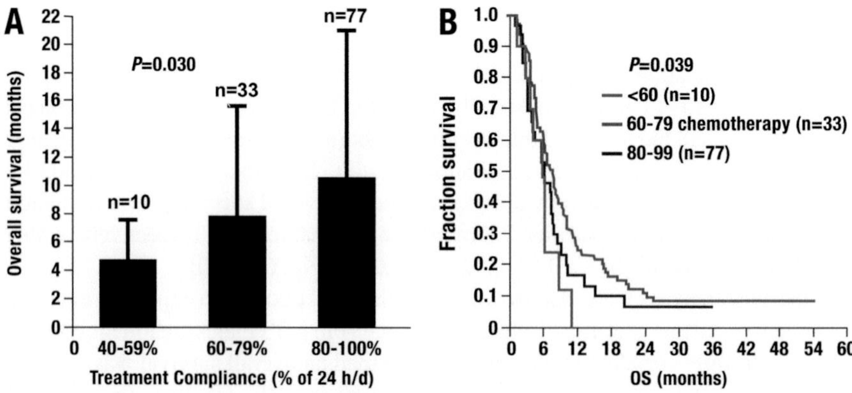


**Fig. 6.6** *Post hoc* analysis of TTFields treatment compliance and survival in the EF-11 trial. (**A**) Spearman rank correlation between treatment compliance and mean OS showed a correlation coefficient of 0.175 (one-sided $p=0.030$). (**B**) Kaplan-Meier OS curves stratified according to compliance. There was a trend for longer median OS with better compliance, with median OS of 5.8 months for <60 % compliance ($n=10$), 6.0 months for 60–79 % compliance ($n=33$), and 7.7 months for 80–99 % compliance ($n=77$) (log-rank test for trend, $\chi^2$ $p=0.039$). *OS* overall survival, $\chi^2$ chi-square. From Kanner et al. *Post Hoc* analyses of intention-to-treat population in phase III comparison of NovoTTF-100A™ system versus best physician's choice chemotherapy. Semin Oncol. 41:S25-S34, 2014. With permission from Elsevier

tively, with a hazard ratio of 0.64 (95 % CI 0.41–0.99) ($p=0.045$) [30] (Fig. 6.7). There was no difference in survival between TTFields monotherapy and non-bevacizumab chemotherapy ($n=84$): median overall survival 6.6 months versus 6.6 months, with a hazard ratio of 0.92 (95 % CI 0.68–1.24) ($p=0.586$) [30].

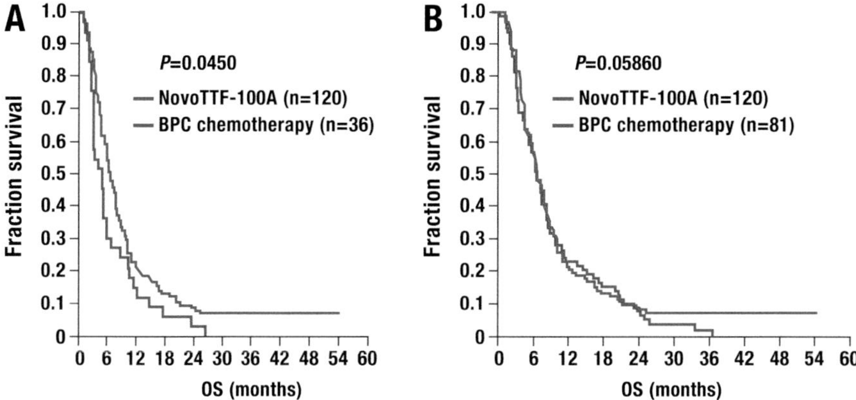


**Fig. 6.7** *Post hoc* analysis of TTFields monotherapy versus bevacizumab and non-bevacizumab treatments. Overall comparison of Kaplan-Meier OS curves for ITT population with recurrent glioblastoma treated with TTFields monotherapy ($n=120$) versus (**A**) bevacizumab ($n=36$) or (**B**) non-bevacizumab ($n=81$) chemotherapy. *ITT* intent to treat, *OS* overall survival. From Kanner et al. Post Hoc analyses of intention-to-treat population in phase III comparison of NovoTTF-100A™ system versus best physician's choice chemotherapy. Semin Oncol. 41:S25-S34, 2014. With permission from Elsevier

## Conclusions

The Optune® device delivered TTFields as treatment for recurrent glioblastoma in the pilot study and the EF-11 phase III trial. In the smaller pilot study, favorable survival characteristics were observed in 10 participants treated with TTFields. However, the subsequent phase III EF-11 trial showed only comparable efficacy when TTFields monotherapy was compared to Best Physician's Choice chemotherapy. The U.S. Food and Drug Administration nevertheless approved the use of the device in this population on April 8, 2011, based on the comparable efficacy, superior safety profile, and a better quality of life. Later, multiple *post hoc* analyses were performed and revealed a number of important findings that explains the discrepancy between the robust data from the pilot study and the results in the phase III trial. First, 27 (23 %) subjects did not receive a complete cycle of TTFields monotherapy and, when these subjects were removed from comparison with those treated with chemotherapy in the modified intent-to-treat analysis, TTFields were found to be superior to chemotherapy. Indeed, TTFields treatment compliance of 75 % or greater was later found to be significantly correlated with overall survival in the participants. Second, a higher dexamethasone dosage (>4.1 mg/day) used by some of the subjects had a negative effect on their survival outcome regardless of treatment with either TTFields or chemotherapy. Therefore, adhering to the recommended treatment compliance and minimizing the amount of daily dexamethasone intake will likely improve the outcome of patients treated with TTFields.

## References

1. Bleeker FE, Molenaar RJ, Leenstra S, et al. Recent advances in the molecular understanding of glioblastoma. J Neurooncol. 2012;108:11–27.
2. Ohgaki H, Dessen P, Jourde B, Hortsmann S, Nishikawa T, Di Patre PL, et al. Genetic pathways to glioblastoma: a population-based study. Cancer Res. 2004;64:6892–9.
3. Macdonald DR, Casino TL, Schold Jr SC, Cairncross JG. Response criteria for phase II studies of supratentorial malignant glioma. J Clin Oncol. 1990;8:1277–80.
4. Wen PY, Macdonald DR, Reardon DA, Cloughesy TF, Sorensen G, Galanis E, et al. Updated response assessment criteria for high-grade gliomas: Response Assessment in Neuro-Oncology working group. J Clin Oncol. 2010;28:1963–72.
5. Wong ET, Brem S. Antiangiogenesis treatment for glioblastoma multiforme: challenges and opportunities. J Natl Compr Canc Netw. 2008;6:515–22.
6. De Wit MCY, de Bruin HG, Eijkenboom W, Sillevis Smitt PAE, van den Bent MJ. Immediate post-radiotherapy changes in malignant glioma can mimic tumor progression. Neurology. 2004;63:535–7.
7. Wong ET. Tumor growth, invasion, and angiogenesis in malignant gliomas. J Neurooncol. 2006;77:295–6.
8. Wong ET, Hess KR, Gleason MJ, Jaeckle KA, Kyritsis AP, Prados MD, et al. Outcomes and prognostic factors in recurrent glioma patients enrolled onto phase II clinical trials. J Clin Oncol. 1999;17:2572–8.
9. Bloch O, Han SH, Cha S, Sun MZ, Aghi MK, McDermott MW, et al. Impact of extent of resection for recurrent glioblastoma on overall survival. J Neurosurg. 2012;117:1032–8.
10. Brem H, Piantadosi S, Burger PC, Walker M, Selker R, Vick NA, et al. Placebo-controlled trial of safety and efficacy of intraoperative controlled delivery by biodegradable polymers of chemotherapy for recurrent gliomas. Lancet. 1995;345:1008–12.
11. Shaw E, Scott C, Souhami L, Dinapoli R, Kline R, Loeffler J, et al. Single dose radiosurgical treatment of recurrent previously irradiated primary brain tumors and brain metastases: final report of RTOG 90-05. Int J Radiat Oncol Biol Phys. 2000;47:291–8.
12. Biswas T, Okunieff P, Schell MC, Smudzin T, Pilcher WH, Bakos RS, et al. Stereotactic radiosurgery for glioblastoma: retrospective analysis. Radiat Oncol. 2009;4:11.
13. Reardon DA, Herndon JE, Peters KB, Desjardins A, Coan A, Lou E, et al. Bevacizumab continuation beyond initial bevacizumab progression among recurrent glioblastoma patients. Br J Cancer. 2012;107:1481–7.
14. Iwamoto FM, Fine HA. Bevacizumab for malignant glioma. Arch Neurol. 2010;67:285–8.
15. Kirson ED, Gurvich Z, Schneiderman R, Dekel E, Itzhaki A, Wasserman Y, et al. Disruption of cancer cell replication by alternating electric fields. Cancer Res. 2004;64:3288–95.
16. Gera N, Yang A, Holtzman TS, Lee SX, Wong ET, Swanson KD. Tumor treating fields perturb the localization of septins and cause aberrant mitotic exit. PLoS One. 2015;10:e0125269.
17. Lee SX, Wong E, Swanson K. Disruption of cell division within anaphase by tumor treating electric fields (TTFields) leads to immunogenic cell death. Neuro-Oncology. 2013;15 Suppl 3:iii66–7.
18. Felder CE, Prilusky J, Silman I, Sussman JL. A server and database for dipole moments of proteins. Nucleic Acids Res. 2007;35:W512–21.
19. Sirajuddin M, Farkasovsky M, Hauer F, Kuhlmann D, Macara IG, Weyand M, et al. Structural insight into filament formation by mammalian septins. Nature. 2007;449:311–5.
20. Yvon AM, Wadsworth P, Jordan MA. Taxol suppresses dynamics of individual microtubules in living human tumor cells. Mol Biol Cell. 1999;10:947–59.
21. Kirson ED, Dbaly V, Tovarys F, Vymazal J, Soustiel JF, Itzhaki A, et al. Alternating electric fields arrest cell proliferation in animal tumor models and human brain tumors. Proc Natl Acad Sci U S A. 2007;104:10152–7.

22. Rulseh AM, Keller J, Klener J, Sroubek J, Dbaly V, Syrucek M, et al. Long-term survival of patients suffering from glioblastoma multiforme treated with tumor treating fields. World J Surg Oncol. 2012;10:220.
23. Stupp R, Wong ET, Kanner AA, Steinberg D, Engelhard H, Heidecke V, et al. NovoTTF-100A versus physician's choice chemotherapy in recurrent glioblastoma: a randomized phase III trial of a novel treatment modality. Eur J Cancer. 2012;48:2192–202.
24. Lacouture ME, Davis ME, Elzinga G, Butowski N, Tran D, Villano JL, et al. Characterization and management of dermatologic adverse events with the NovoTTF-100A System, a novel anti-mitotic electric field device for the treatment of recurrent glioblastoma. Semin Oncol. 2014;41 Suppl 4:S1–14.
25. Wong ET, Lok E, Swanson KD, Gautam S, Engelhard HH, Lieberman F, et al. Response assessment of NovoTTF-100A versus best physician's choice chemotherapy in recurrent glioblastoma. Cancer Med. 2014;3:592–602.
26. Wong ET, Lok E, Gautam S, Swanson KD. Dexamethasone exerts profound immunologic interference on treatment efficacy for recurrent glioblastoma. Br J Cancer. 2015;113:232–41.
27. Back MF, Ang EL, Ng WH, See SJ, Lim CC, Chan SP, et al. Improved median survival for glioblastoma multiforme following introduction of adjuvant temozolomide chemotherapy. Ann Acad Med Singapore. 2007;36:338–42.
28. Rutz HP, Hofer S, Peghini PE, Gutteck-Amsler U, Rentsch K, Meier-Abt PJ, et al. Avoiding glucocorticoid administration in a neurooncological case. Cancer Biol Ther. 2005;4:1186–9.
29. Pitter KL, Tamagno I, Alikhanyan K, Hosni-Ahmed A, Pattwell SS, Donnola S, et al. Corticosteroids compromise survival in glioblastoma. Brain. 2016;139:1458–1471.
30. Kanner AA, Wong ET, Villano JL, Ram Z, et al. Post hoc analyses of intention-to-treat population in phase III comparison of NovoTTF-100A System versus best physician's choice chemotherapy. Semin Oncol. 2014;41:S25–34.

# Chapter 7
# Tumor Treating Fields in Clinical Practice with Emphasis on PRiDe Registry

**Jacob Ruzevick, Eric T. Wong, and Maciej M. Mrugala**

Glioblastoma (GBM) is the most common primary malignant brain tumor in adults and is universally associated with a poor prognosis. Despite aggressive treatments consisting of maximal neurosurgical resection, chemotherapy, and radiation, patient outcomes remain poor with a median time to recurrence of approximately 7 months and a median overall survival of about 15 months [1, 2]. Following recurrence, the median progression-free survival and overall survival are approximately 9 weeks and 25 weeks, respectively [3]. The drug commonly used to treat patients with recurrent GBM is bevacizumab, which gained accelerated approval from the U.S. Food and Drug Administration in 2009 after two single-arm studies demonstrated a high radiologic response rate that was associated with improved clinical outcome [4–6]. While new drugs, such as small molecule tyrosine kinase inhibitors, monoclonal antibodies, and immune therapies, are rapidly changing the landscape of treatment options for GBM, this tumor inevitably develops resistance to systemic therapies. Therefore, multimodality treatment approach is critical for continued improvement of patient outcomes.

J. Ruzevick, M.D.
Department of Neurological Surgery, University of Washington
and Fred Hutchinson Cancer Research Center, Seattle, WA, USA

E.T. Wong, M.D.
Division of Neuro-Oncology, Department of Neurology, Beth Israel Deaconess
Medical Center, Boston, MA, USA

Department of Physics, University of Massachusetts in Lowell, Lowell, MA 01854, USA

M.M. Mrugala, M.D., Ph.D., M.P.H. (✉)
Department of Neurological Surgery, University of Washington
and Fred Hutchinson Cancer Research Center, Seattle, WA, USA

Department of Neurology, University of Washington
and Fred Hutchinson Cancer Research Center, Seattle, WA, USA

Department of Medicine, University of Washington
and Fred Hutchinson Cancer Research Center, Seattle, WA, USA
e-mail: mmrugala@uw.edu



E.T. Wong (ed.), *Alternating Electric Fields Therapy in Oncology*,
DOI 10.1007/978-3-319-30576-9_7

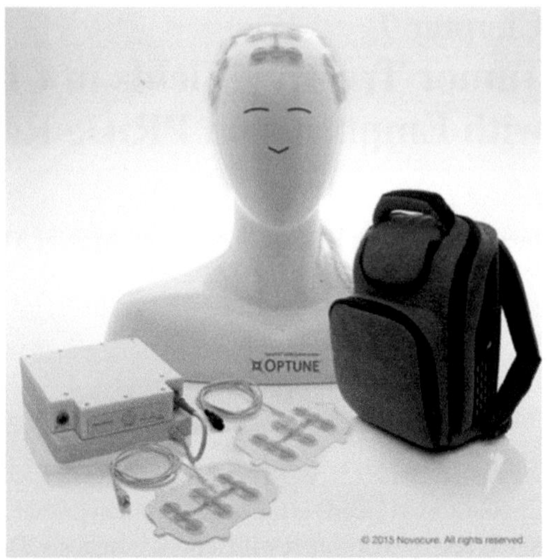


**Fig. 7.1** The Optune® device is comprised of transducer arrays that are placed on the scalp and connected to the field generator. This portable system is used in 4-week cycles with optimal results seen when compliance exceeds 75 % daily use (18 hours a day or more). Courtesy of Novocure

The Optune® device (Novocure Ltd., Haifa, Israel) was approved by the U.S. Food and Drug Administration in 2011 for use in patients with recurrent GBM [7]. The system is a portable, noninvasive device that delivers medium frequency (200 kHz) alternating electric fields, also known as Tumor Treating Fields (TTFields), directly to the tumor bed and peri-tumoral tissues. The unit can be carried in a compact backpack or used as a stationary unit with transducer arrays placed directly on the patient's scalp (Fig. 7.1). Unlike chemotherapeutics, which can exert anti-neoplastic activity long after dosing, TTFields therapy has no half-life, requiring that the device be worn continually in order to produce a beneficial anti-mitotic effect. A single "cycle" of TTFields therapy is 4 weeks of near continuous usage as this was shown to be the time course necessary for the electric fields to exert therapeutic effects on GBM [8]. The approval in the recurrent GBM population was based on the EF-11 phase III trial results in which 237 subjects were randomized in a 1:1 ratio to receive TTFields monotherapy versus best physician's choice chemotherapy [9]. The trial demonstrated that patient survival from TTFields was comparable to chemotherapy, while adverse event and quality of life analyses favored TTFields.

Clinical trials data may not always be representative of patient treatment outcome in a routine clinical practice environment. There are a number of reasons for that. First, upon trial entry, subjects must possess prespecified clinical characteristics that real-world patient may not have. As a result, trial subjects typically have better neurologic function, higher performance status, and fewer medical comorbidities, all of which may enable participants in the trial to benefit more from the new treatment. Second, the U.S. Food and Drug Administration must strike a fine balance between providing the public rapid access to new treatments for deadly diseases and requiring comprehensive data on their benefits and risks. This action sometimes results in the reversal of prior accelerated approval decisions for oncologic therapies. For example, approvals for bevacizumab in breast cancer and gefitinib for non-small cell lung cancer was reversed after additional efficacy data showed no benefit [10–14]. Furthermore, after the accelerated approval of bevacizumab for recurrent GBM, two large-scale randomized phase III trials testing this drug in newly diagnosed patients did not show survival benefit [15, 16]. Therefore, bevacizumab's indication for GBM is also at risk of withdrawal. Lastly, oncologists and other medical practitioners may have inherent beliefs, either conscious or subconscious, that may bias them toward not adapting the new treatment despite available evidence [17]. Therefore, post-approval registry may provide valuable information on the pattern of usage and the efficacy of new therapy in the real-world setting.

## Real World Clinical Experience with Tumor Treating Fields

The efficacy of TTFields in recurrent GBM has been shown in prospective studies with the most important one being a phase III randomized clinical trial comparing TTFields monotherapy to physician's best choice of chemotherapy (the EF-11 trial). A summary of clinical studies of TTFields in GBM is shown in Table 7.1. The results of these studies are discussed in Chapter 6.

**Table 7.1** Baseline patient characteristics in PRiDe and EF-11 trial.

| Patient characteristics | | PRiDe TTFields therapy ($n=457$) | EF-11 TTFields therapy ($n=120$) | EF-11 chemotherapy ($n=117$) |
|---|---|---|---|---|
| Age (years) | Median (range) | 55 (18–86) | 54 (24–80) | 54 (29–74) |
| Gender | Male | 67.6 % | 77 % | 62 % |
| | Female | 32.4 % | 23 % | 38 % |
| KPS | Median (range) | 80 (10–100) | 80 (50–100) | 80 (50–100) |
| | 10–60 | 19.0 % | NA | NA |
| | 70–80 | 46.6 % | NA | NA |
| | 90–100 | 30.9 % | NA | NA |
| | Unknown | 3.5 % | NA | NA |
| Recurrence | Median (range) | 2 (1–5) | 2 (1–5) | 2 (1–4) |
| | First | 33.3 % | 9 % | 15 % |
| | Second | 26.9 % | 48 % | 46 % |
| | Third to fifth | 27.4 % | 43 % | 39 % |
| | Unknown | 12.5 % | 0 % | 0 % |
| Prior treatments | Bevacizumab | 55.1 % | 19 % | 18 % |
| | RT+temozolomide | 77.9 % | 86 % | 82 % |
| | Debulking surgery | 63.9 % | 79 % | 85 % |
| | Carmustine wafers | 3.7 % | NA | NA |

*KPS* Karnofsky performance status, *NA* not available, *RT* radiotherapy

## *Patient Registry Dataset (PRiDe)*

As the Optune® device became available after U.S. Food and Drug Administration approval in clinical neuro-oncology practices, the PRiDe registry was set up in late 2011 to collect data on patients who were treated with TTFields for recurrent GBM [18]. From October 2011 thru November 2013, data on 457 patients were captured from 91 neuro-oncology centers or oncology practices certified to administer the device in the United States. All patients provided informed consent to allow their protected health information to be used for this registry. They also had a histologically confirmed diagnosis of GBM and recurrence was defined radiologically according to the Macdonald criteria [19]. Unlike patients in the pivotal phase III study, there were no exclusions based on previous radiation or chemotherapy regimens. Baseline clinical characteristics of patients were tabulated by chart review. Centralized collection of compliance data, which contain the cumulative amount of time therapy was delivered to the patient, were obtained by Novocure from an internal log file downloaded from each device. Compliance data was only available for two-thirds of participants because Novocure only started collecting this information centrally in January of 2013. Patient compliance was calculated as the average percentage of each day or a 24-hour period that the device was delivering TTFields. Prognostic factors such as age, Karnofsky performance status, debulking surgeries, the number of prior GBM recurrences, and prior bevacizumab use were captured for analysis. Adverse events were graded according to the National Cancer Institute Common Terminology Criteria for Adverse Events (CTCAE). Patient survival information was captured using the United States Social Security Death Date Registry and obituaries.

There are a number of differences between participants in PRiDe and the TTFields monotherapy cohort in the EF-11 trial [9, 18]. First, patients who received the device in PRiDe were not restricted to TTFields treatment only. However, information on combined use of the device with other chemotherapies and/or bevacizumab, which was at the discretion of the treating physician, was not captured. In addition, some of the patients included in PRiDe could have been exhibiting pseudoprogression following combined chemotherapy and radiation, a known radiographic phenomenon that typically occurs within the first 12 weeks after treatment [20]. Second, as mentioned above, compliance data were captured from only about two-thirds of the patients. Lastly, PRiDe did not capture data on quality of life measures. Although these differences may make comparisons between the two groups of patients challenging, PRiDe nonetheless offers a unique opportunity to examine treatment efficacy and toxicities of the Optune® device in a real-world practice environment.

## *Patient Characteristics and Survival Differences Between PRiDe and EF-11*

Baseline patient characteristics from PRiDe and comparison to the two cohorts in EF-11 are shown in Table 7.2. Among the 457 participants in PRiDe, the average age was 55 years (range 18–86) and approximately a third of them were women.

**Table 7.2** Summary of clinical trials in GBM involving TTFields.

| Study | *n* | Pathology | Study treatment | Median overall survival | | Progression-free survival | |
|---|---|---|---|---|---|---|---|
| | | | | TTFields | Chemotherapy | TTFields | Chemotherapy |
| Kirson et al. 2007 [24] | 10 | Recurrent GBM | TTFields only | 14.4 months | – | 6.0 months | – |
| Stupp et al. 2012 [8] | 237 | Recurrent GBM | TTFields vs best physician's choice chemotherapy | 6.6 months | 6.0 months | 2.2 months | 2.1 months |
| Mrugala et al. 2014 [18] | 457 | Recurrent GBM | TTFields ± chemotherapy | 9.6 months | | | |

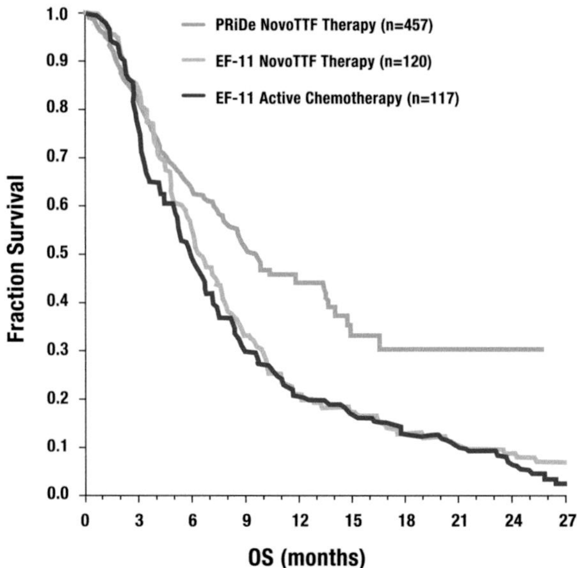


**Fig. 7.2** Kaplan-Meier estimate of overall survival (OS) curves for patients with recurrent GBM treated with TTFields in PRiDe versus those received TTFields monotherapy or best physician's choice chemotherapy in the EF-11 trial. From Mrugala et al. Clinical practice experience with NovoTTF-100A™ system for glioblastoma: The Patient Registry Dataset (PRiDe). Semin Oncol. 41 Suppl 6: S4-S13, 2014. Elsevier

The median Karnofsky performance status was 80 (range 10–100). The median number of GBM recurrences prior to entry into PRiDe was 2 (range 1–5). Fifty-five percent of patients had previously been treated with bevacizumab, which is a greater number of patients than the 19 % in the EF-11 TTFields monotherapy arm. Approximately 78 % of them had received previous radiation and chemotherapy while 63 % had debulking surgery.

A major finding in PRiDe is that the median overall survival in patients treated in clinical practice was improved as compared to TTFields monotherapy in the EF-11 phase III trial, 9.6 months versus 6.6 months respectively (Table 7.2 and Fig. 7.2), even though these two groups are not statistically comparable [18, 21, 22]. This favorable survival trend also extended out to the 2-year timeline with a respective survival rate of 30 % versus 9 % (Table 7.3) [18]. The improved survival among the patients in PRiDe may be due to a greater number (33 %) starting treatment at the first recurrence, and fewer (27 %) receiving it at third to fifth recurrences, as compared to only 9 % and 43 % respectively in EF-11. While the patients included in the PRiDe were more diverse and heterogeneous, they received a significantly longer duration of treatment as compared to those treated in EF-11, 4.1 months versus 2.3 months respectively [18]. Approximately 10 % of those patients in the PRiDe continued on TTFields treatment for at least 2 years.

**Table 7.3** One- and 2-year overall survival rates for patients with recurrent glioblastoma multiforme treated with TTFields therapy in PRiDe and EF-11 trial, and with best physician's choice chemotherapy in the EF-11 trial

| Endpoint | PRiDe TTFields therapy ($n = 457$) | EF-11 TTFields therapy ($n = 120$) | EF-11 chemotherapy ($n = 117$) |
|---|---|---|---|
| 1-Year survival | 44 % | 20 % | 20 % |
| 2-Year survival | 30 % | 9 % | 7 % |

**Table 7.4** Summary of dermatologic adverse events in clinical studies involving TTFields.

| Study | $n$ | Pathology | Study treatment | Dermatologic AE |
|---|---|---|---|---|
| Kirson et al. 2007 [24] | 10 | Recurrent GBM | TTFields only | 90 % |
| Stupp et al. 2012 [9] | 237 | Recurrent GBM | TTFields vs. best physician's choice chemotherapy | Grade I/II: 16 %<br>Grade III/IV: 3 % |
| Mrugala et al. 2014 [18] | 457 | Recurrent GBM | TTFields ± chemotherapy | 24 % |

## *No Unexpected Adverse Events in PRiDe*

The tolerability and safety of TTFields treatment in PRiDe were analyzed and no unexpected adverse events were found when compared to prior trials. The most common device-related side effects were skin reactions, heat sensations, and electric sensations on the scalp associated with the transducer arrays, occurring at a rate of 24 %, 11 %, and 8 %, respectively (Tables 7.4 and 7.5) [18]. Nervous system-related events were the second most common adverse events, and included neurological disorders (10 %), seizures (9 %), and headaches (6 %). Many of the nervous system-associated events were likely associated with the recurrent GBM [18].

## *Prognostic Factors in PRiDe*

A number of prognostic factors were identified in the PRiDe population and they are displayed in Figs. 7.3 and 7.4. Similar to the prospective EF-11 study, compliance ≥75 % was notably associated with improved median overall survival when compared to <75 %, 13.5 months versus 4.0 months, with a hazard ratio of 0.4 (95 % CI 0.3–0.6) ($p < 0.001$, Fig. 7.3) [18]. This finding is consistent with device's mechanism of action in that TTFields disrupt tumor cells during mitosis and the fields have to be present continuously in order to exert its anti-tumor effect. Other favorable prognostic factors included early introduction of therapy and higher Karnofsky performance status (Fig. 7.4) [18]. Patients who failed bevacizumab did not respond as well, most likely because of the more extensive infiltration of the brain by recurrent glioblastoma. Debulking surgery that was performed prior to the application of the device did not influence patient survival (Fig. 7.4).

**Table 7.5** Adverse events in patients with recurrent glioblastoma treated with TTFields in PRiDe.

| Adverse event | Percentage of patients PRiDe ($n$=457) |
|---|---|
| Skin reaction | 24.3 |
| Heat sensation | 11.3 |
| Neurological disorder | 10.4 |
| Seizure | 8.9 |
| Electric sensation | 7.7 |
| Headache | 5.7 |
| Pain/discomfort | 4.7 |
| Fall | 3.9 |
| Psychiatric disorder | 2.9 |
| Gastrointestinal disorder | 2.9 |
| Fatigue | 2.5 |
| Vascular disorder | 1.6 |
| Weakness | 1.4 |
| Infections | 1.4 |
| Eye disorder | 1.3 |

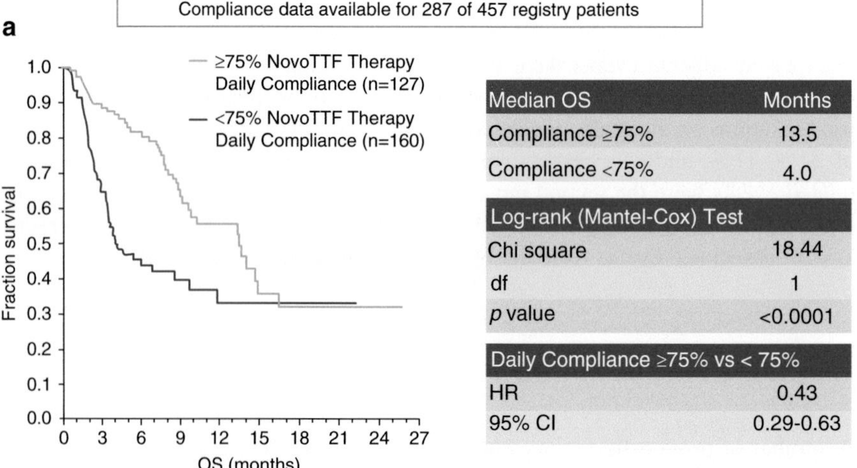


**Fig. 7.3** Treatment compliance with TTFields. (**a**) Results from PRiDe with respect to overall survival by daily compliance, dichotomized according to ≥75 % versus <75 %, with TTFields therapy for recurrent GBM. (**b**) Representative compliance report generated after a cycle of TTFields therapy. (**a**) From Mrugala et al. Clinical practice experience with NovoTTF-100A™ system for glioblastoma: The Patient Registry Dataset (PRiDe). Semin Oncol. 41 Suppl: S4-S13, 2014. Elsevier. (**b**) Courtesy of Novocure

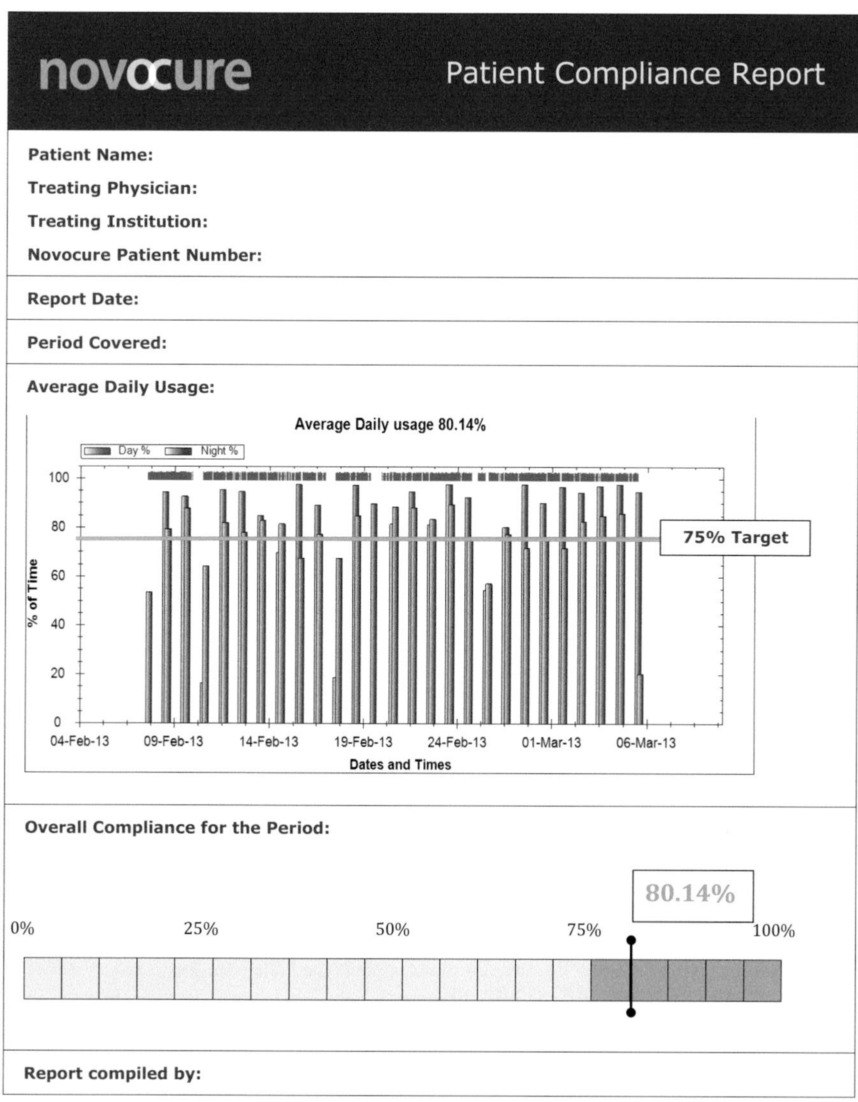


**Fig. 7.3** (continued)

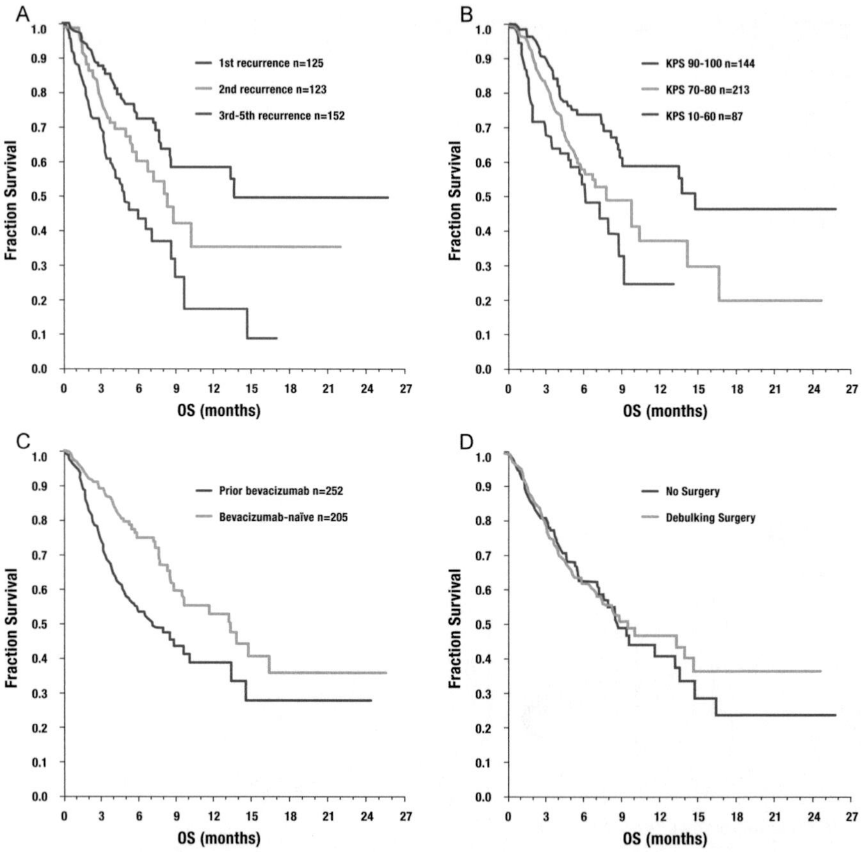


**Fig. 7.4** Kaplan-Meier estimate of overall survival curves for patients with recurrent GBM treated with TTFields in PRiDe according to (**A**) recurrence number, (**B**) Karnofsky performance status, (**C**) prior bevacizumab use, and (**D**) prior debulking surgery. From Mrugala et al. Clinical practice experience with NovoTTF-100A™ system for glioblastoma: The Patient Registry Dataset (PRiDe). Semin Oncol. 41 Suppl 6: pp S4-S13, 2014. Elsevier

## Special Clinical Considerations for Patients Treated with Tumor Treating Fields

One unique situation to consider in patients with GBM who might be candidates for TTFields therapy is the presence of intracranial hardware, such as shunts for cerebrospinal fluid diversion. While shunts with programmable valves were part of the exclusion criteria for EF-11, Mrugala et al. [23] reported that TTFields were used safely in a single patient with a nonprogrammable ventriculo-peritoneal shunt (Fig. 7.5). Since cerebrospinal fluid diversion is common in patients operated on for intracranial tumors, additional reports of the use of nonprogrammable shunts are needed to establish their safety in the setting of TTFields

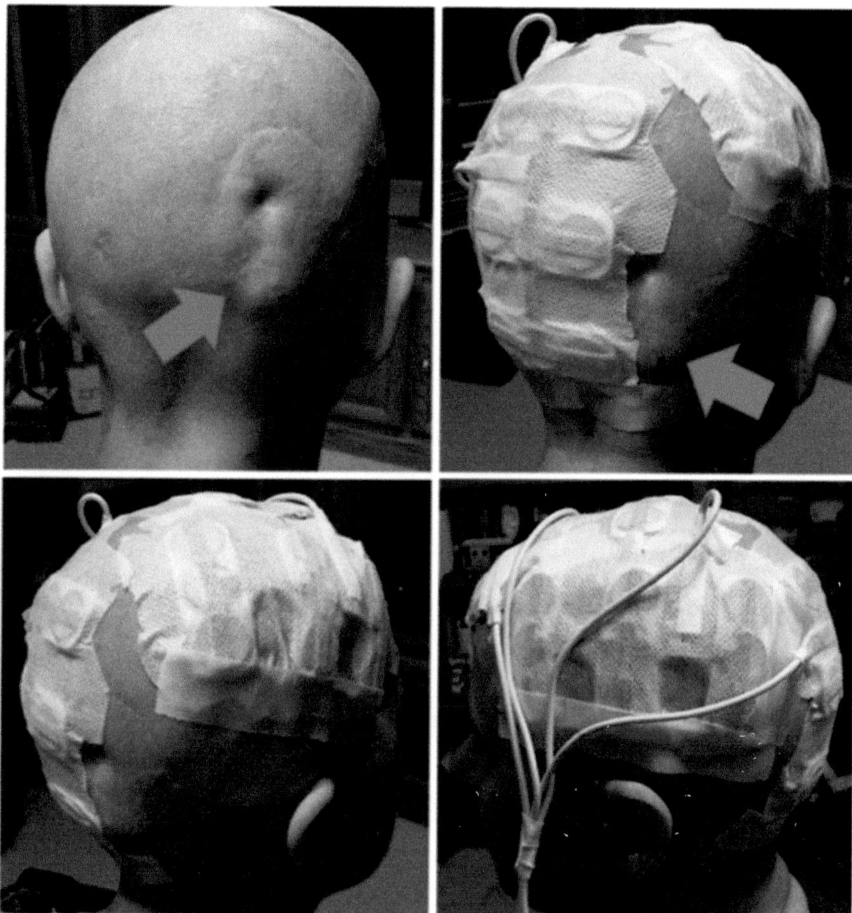

**Fig. 7.5** The Optune® device was successfully utilized in a patient with ventriculo-peritoneal shunt and nonprogrammable valve. *Arrows* identify the valve in relationship to the treatment arrays. The patient used TTFields for over 12 months and experienced no complication.

application. Data pertaining to this issue are being actively collected and will be published in the near future.

Intensity of the electrical fields being applied to the tumor and the surrounding tissues heavily depends on the positioning of the treatment arrays on the scalp. In general, the closer the arrays are to each other, the higher the intensity of the fields and consequently greater efficacy of the anti-mitotic activity from the treatment. To identify the optimal positioning of the transducer arrays, the NovoTAL™ (transducer array layout) system was developed (Fig. 7.6). This system inputs magnetic resonance imaging of a gender-specific head morphology, tumor location, and size to optimize the intensity of TTFields directed at the tumor. The NovoTAL™ system, approved by the U.S. Food and Drug Administration for clinical use, allows treating physicians to generate treatment maps and adjust them accordingly during treatment when tumor-specific parameters change.

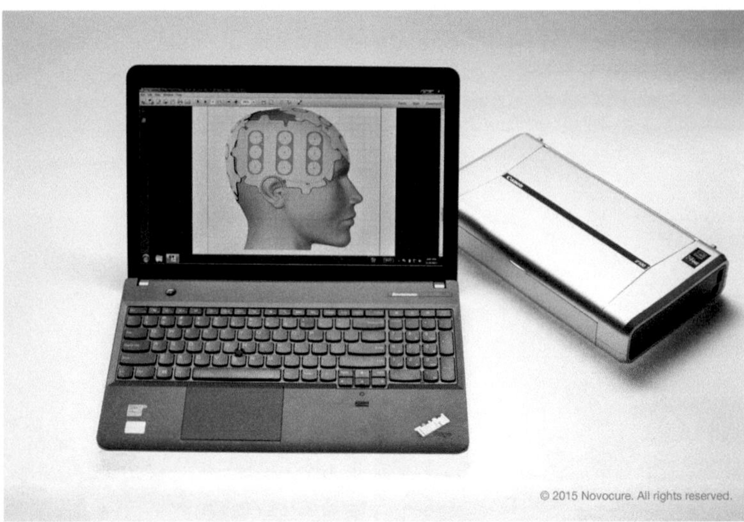


**Fig. 7.6** NovoTAL™ system allows physicians to create treatment maps and customize TTFields therapy. The intensity of the electric fields can be modulated and optimized by changing the location of the transducer arrays. Courtesy of Novocure

## Dermatologic Side Effects of Tumor Treating Fields Therapy

Hematologic and gastrointestinal toxicities frequently seen in association with chemotherapeutics are not encountered with TTFields therapy. Given the mode of administration through the direct placement of treatment arrays on the skin, dermatologic complications were the most commonly seen side effect in all reported clinical studies [9, 18]. Skin-related complications resulting from the use of the device include dermatitis, erosions, infections, and ulcers. Most of these complications are likely a result of mechanical trauma from repeated application of arrays, poor wound healing, and potentially combination treatment with chemotherapeutics. Dermatologic complications of TTFields treatment will be discussed in detail in Chapter 9.

## Conclusions

GBM is one of the most difficult cancers to treat and surgical resection, radiation, and systemic chemotherapy do not offer a cure. TTFields represent a novel and unique treatment method. This anti-mitotic device is externally worn on the scalp and is not associated with the typical systemic side effects seen with chemotherapy. The pivotal randomized phase III clinical trial showed a median overall survival of 6.6 months in recurrent GBM subjects, similar to what can be achieved with standard chemotherapies but with fewer side effects. PRiDe is a large registry of 457 patients with recurrent glioblastoma treated with TTFields therapy in routine clinical practice after approval by the U.S. Food and Drug Administration in 2011. Even though this registry cannot be directly compared to the randomized prospective trial, outcome data from this dataset provide an important adjunct in assessing the true efficacy of the device. Key findings from PRiDe include a significantly longer overall survival as compared to the TTFields monotherapy cohort in the EF-11 phase III trial and excellent tolerability. Favorable prognostic factors include good treatment compliance and higher Karnofsky performance status. Moreover, data from PRiDe indicate that earlier introduction (at first progression) of treatment may result in improved outcomes in recurrent GBM and that bevacizumab-naïve patients benefit from TTFields more than patients previously treated. Patient compliance with this continuous anti-cancer therapy is critical as increased usage (18 hours per day or more) is associated with improved survival. The reasons for the difference in outcomes between the EF-11 clinical trial and the PRiDe dataset are not fully understood. Several factors, discussed above, might have played a role and these include combination therapies and potential pseudoprogression issue in PRiDe, as well as selection bias towards worse performing subjects in the EF-11 trial. Nevertheless, patients in PRiDe collectively appear to perform better than those enrolled in EF-11 and this dataset offers an important view of TTFields treatment efficacy in the real-world setting.

The Optune® device can be safely and effectively used in the clinical practice setting after appropriate training and credentialing process is completed. The NovoTAL™ platform allows physicians to customize therapy to the individual patient and adjust treatment planning during the course of therapy. Ultimately, physician experience accumulated during clinical practice will improve the clinical application of this device.

## References

1. Stupp R, Mason WP, van den Bent MJ, Weller M, Fisher B, Taphoorn MJB, et al. Radiotherapy plus concomitant and adjuvant temozolomide for glioblastoma. N Engl J Med. 2005;352:987–96.
2. Stupp R, Hegi ME, Mason WP, van den Bent MJ, Taphoorn MJB, Janzer RC, et al. Effects of radiotherapy with concomitant and adjuvant temozolomide versus radiotherapy alone on survival in glioblastoma in a randomised phase III study: 5-year analysis of the EORTC-NCIC trial. Lancet Oncol. 2009;10:459–66.
3. Wong ET, Hess KR, Gleason MJ, Jaeckle KA, Kyritsis AP, Prados MD, et al. Outcomes and prognostic factors in recurrent glioma patients enrolled onto phase II clinical trials. J Clin Oncol. 1999;17:2572–8.
4. http://www.fda.gov/NewsEvents/Newsroom/PressAnnouncements/ucm152295.htm.
5. Friedman HS, Prados MD, Wen PY, Mikkelsen T, Schiff D, Abrey LE, et al. Bevacizumab alone and in combination with irinotecan in recurrent glioblastoma. J Clin Oncol. 2009;27:4733–40.
6. Kreisl TN, Kim L, Moore K, Duic P, Royce C, Stroud I, et al. Phase II trial of single-agent bevacizumab followed by bevacizumab plus irinotecan at tumor progression in recurrent glioblastoma. J Clin Oncol. 2009;27:740–5.

7. http://www.fda.gov/NewsEvents/Newsroom/PressAnnouncements/ucm251669.htm.
8. Kirson ED, Wasserman Y, Izhaki A, Mordechovich D, Gurvich Z, Dbaly V, et al. Modeling tumor growth kinetics and its implications for TTFields treatment planning. Neuro-Oncology. 2010;12 Suppl 4:iv48.
9. Stupp R, Wong ET, Kanner AA, Steinberg D, Engelhard H, Heidecke V, et al. NovoTTF-100A versus physician's choice chemotherapy in recurrent glioblastoma: a randomised phase III trial of a novel treatment modality. Eur J Cancer. 2012;48:2192–202.
10. Eichler HG, Pignatti F, Flamion B, Leufkens H, Brenckenridge A. Balancing early market access to new drugs with the need for benefit/risk data: a mounting dilemma. Nat Rev Drug Discov. 2008;7:818–26.
11. Lenzer J. FDA committee votes to withdraw bevacizumab for breast cancer. BMJ. 2011;343:d4244.
12. http://www.fda.gov/NewsEvents/Newsroom/PressAnnouncements/ucm280536.htm.
13. Senderowicz AM, Pfaff O. Similarities and differences in the oncology drug approval process between FDA and European Union with emphasis on in vitro companion diagnostics. Clin Cancer Res. 2014;20:1445–52.
14. https://www.federalregister.gov/articles/2012/04/25/2012-9944/astrazeneca-pharmaceuticals-lp-withdrawal-of-approval-of-a-new-drug-application-for-iressa.
15. Gilbert MR, Dignam JJ, Armstrong TS, Wefel JS, Blumenthal DT, et al. A randomized trial of bevacizumab for newly diagnosed glioblastoma. N Engl J Med. 2014;370:699–708.
16. Chinot OL, Wick W, Mason W, Henriksson R, Saran F, Nishkawa R, et al. Bevacizumab plus radiotherapy-temozolomide for newly diagnosed glioblastoma. N Engl J Med. 2014;370: 709–22.
17. Tognoni G, Alli C, Avanzini F, Bettelli G, Colombo F, Corso R, et al. Randomised clinical trials in general practice: lessons from a failure. BMJ. 1991;303:969–71.
18. Mrugala MM, Engelhard HH, Dinh Tran D, Kew Y, Cavaliere R, Villano JL, et al. Clinical practice experience with NovoTTF-100A™ system for glioblastoma: the Patient Registry Dataset (PRiDe). Semin Oncol. 2014;41 Suppl 6:S4–13.
19. Macdonald DR, Casino TL, Schold Jr SC, Cairncross JG. Response criteria for phase II studies of supratentorial malignant glioma. J Clin Oncol. 1990;8:1277–80.
20. Taal W, Brandsma D, de Bruin HG, Bromberg JE, Swaak-Kragten AT, Smitt PA, et al. Incidence of early pseudo-progression in a cohort of malignant glioma patients treated with chemoirradiation with temozolomide. Cancer. 2008;113:405–10.
21. Wong ET, Englehard HH, Tran DD, Kew Y, Mrugala MM, Cavaliere R, et al. NovoTTF-100A alternating electric fields therapy for recurrent glioblastoma: an analysis of patient registry data. Can J Neurol Sci. 2014;41:S9.
22. Wong ET, Englehard HH, Tran DD, Kew Y, Mrugala MM, Cavaliere R, et al. An updated analysis of patient registry data on NovoTTF-100A alternating electric fields therapy for recurrent glioblastoma. Neuro-Oncology. 2014;16 Suppl 5:v74.
23. Mrugala MM, Graham CA, Rockhill JK, Silbergeld DL. Novo-TTF 100A System used successfully in a patient with a ventriculo-peritoneal shunt. Neuro-Oncology. 2014;16 Suppl 2:ii101.
24. Kirson ED, Dbalý V, Tovarys F, Vymazal J, Soustiel JF, Itzhaki A, et al. Alternating electric fields arrest cell proliferation in animal tumor models and human brain tumors. Proc Natl Acad Sci U S A. 2007;104:10152–7.

# Chapter 8
# Tumor Treating Fields Therapy for Newly Diagnosed Glioblastoma

**Eric T. Wong and Zvi Ram**

Glioblastoma is a heterogeneous disease. From a molecular perspective, multiple mutations are found in various signal transduction pathways, including those in the canonical phosphoinositol-3-kinase/mitogen-activated protein kinase pathways that regulate growth and survival, the p53 transcription factor that governs senescence and apoptosis, as well as the retinoblastoma/cyclin-dependent kinase regulatory pathway that controls the cell cycle [1]. At least four molecular subtypes of glioblastoma can be characterized at initial diagnosis and defined according to gene expression profiling as proneural, neural, classical, and mesenchymal subtypes [1, 2]. These glioblastoma subtypes have different responsiveness to treatments; patients with classical and mesenchymal characteristics lived longer when treated with intensive radiotherapy and temozolomide while those with the proneural subtype did not [2]. Further complicating the molecular landscape is the multitude of amplified and mutated genes within each tumor cell. For example, amplifications and mutations of multiple receptor tyrosine kinases and other downstream signaling kinases that regulate key cellular processes are found in varying degrees in individual tumor cells, which eventually give rise to subpopulations with more heterogeneous amplifications and mutations [3–5]. Collectively, these inter-tumoral and intra-tumoral heterogeneities, as well as the tendency to acquire additional mutations as a result of cancer evolution or treatment, invariably make glioblastoma very difficult to control.

E.T. Wong, M.D. (✉)
Division of Neuro-Oncology, Department of Neurology, Beth Israel Deaconess Medical Center, Boston, MA, USA

Department of Physics, University of Massachusetts in Lowell, Lowell, MA 01854, USA
e-mail: ewong@bidmc.harvard.edu

Z. Ram, M.D. (✉)
Department of Neurosurgery, Tel Aviv Sourasky Medical Center, Tel Aviv University, Tel Aviv, Israel
e-mail: zviram@tlvmc.gov.il



E.T. Wong (ed.), *Alternating Electric Fields Therapy in Oncology*,
DOI 10.1007/978-3-319-30576-9_8

The clinical behavior of glioblastoma is multifaceted. Tumor growth and proliferation, angiogenesis and invasion are the clinical hallmarks of this disease, but the extent to which each hallmark appears in individual patients is variable [6]. Furthermore, although the glioblastoma is often detected as a solitary mass at initial diagnosis, some are more invasive than others and appear in a gliomatosis fashion [7]. It can also present in a multifocal pattern, either synchronously with the primary tumor or metachronously as additional foci emerge after initial diagnosis and treatment [8]. Whether or not each individual focus is clonally related is unclear. Under rare circumstances, glioblastoma can even metastasize outside the central nervous system, and this is made possible by the presence of circulating tumor cells [9, 10].

The extensive heterogeneity in the glioblastoma's molecular makeup and clinical behavior presents a daunting challenge in constructing effective treatment regimens for this disease. The tumor also co-opts normal physiological processes, such as angiogenesis and immune tolerance, to subserve its own survival and proliferation within the patient. An obvious strategy is to block deranged intra-tumoral processes, such as amplified or mutated receptor tyrosine kinases and other downstream kinases that are targets for small molecule inhibitors or monoclonal antibodies, but none have yet been shown to benefit glioblastoma patients [11, 12]. Strategies that reverse or normalize co-opted physiological processes may have a chance because these processes are probably less disordered and more amendable to intervention. For example, bevacizumab, which normalizes tumor blood vessels, has been shown to prolong progression-free survival but not overall survival in newly diagnosed patients [13–15]. Furthermore, gross total neurosurgical resection of the glioblastoma provides a means of significant cytoreduction. This cytoreduction not only diminishes the intracranial mass effect that may debilitate patients but also reduces the number of heterogeneous cell types that are resistant to subsequent radiation and chemotherapy. In addition, because loss of *Phosphatase and Tensin Homolog (PTEN)* activates glioblastoma-induced immune suppression, reduction of *PTEN* null or mutated tumors can potentially reduce the tumor's ability to evade the immune system [16, 17]. Lastly, dexamethasone has beneficial anti-edema effects in the brain but it also interferes with immune effector functions against the glioblastoma, as shown in past *post hoc* analyses of the EF-11 trial comparing Tumor Treating Fields (TTFields) with chemotherapy and retrospective analysis of patient outcome from radiation treatment [18–20]. Regardless of the etiology, a drop in the $CD4^+$ lymphocyte counts to <200 cell/mm$^3$ is correlated with a poorer survival compared to ≥200 cell/mm$^3$, suggesting that $CD4^+$ count may serve as a marker of immune competence in the glioblastoma population [21]. A dexamethasone dose <4 mg/day probably provides some anti-edema benefit in patients while not interfering with their immune effector function against the glioblastoma [18, 22]. Alternatives to dexamethasone include bevacizumab, celecoxib, and angiotensin receptor blockers [23–26] that are not thought to interfere with the immune system. Taken together, strategies that block co-opted physiological processes by the glioblastoma, as well as those that accentuate the patient's own anti-tumor response, are more likely to be met with success (Fig. 8.1).

TTFields are a new cancer treatment that can interfere with the co-opted cell division machinery and potentiate anti-tumor immune response. Specifically, the

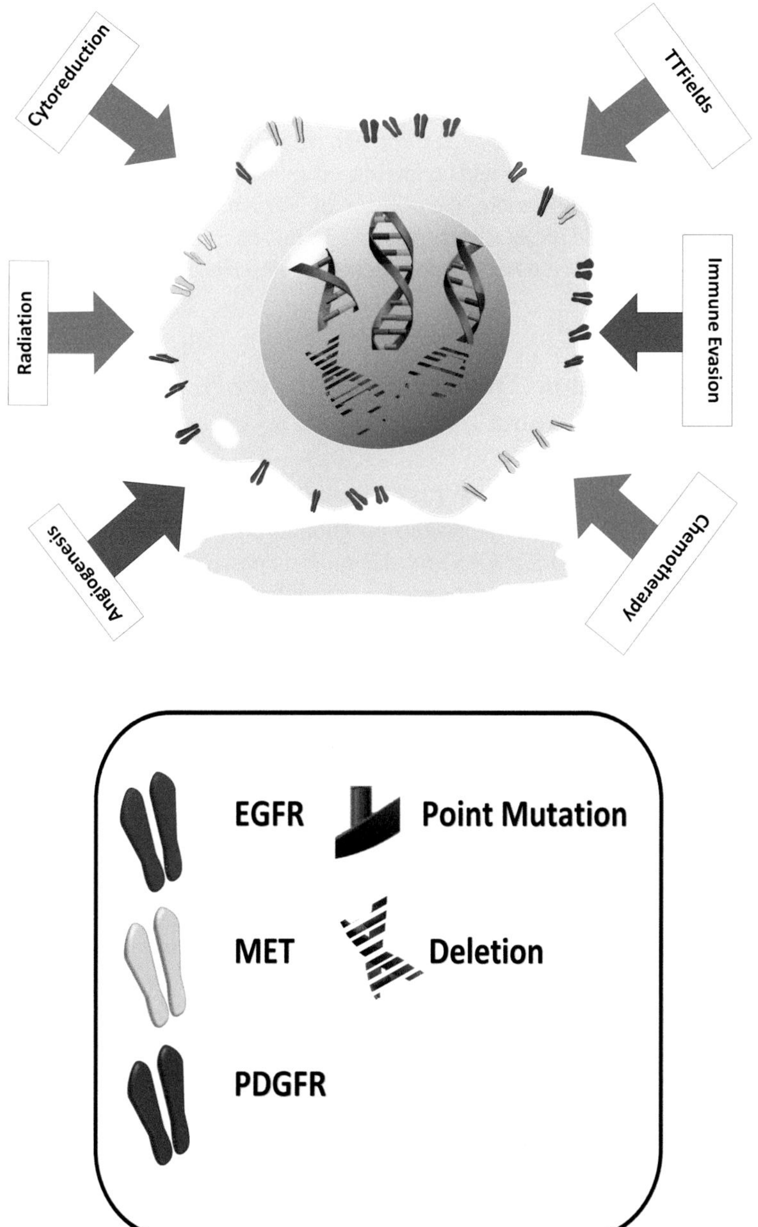


**Fig. 8.1** Glioblastoma tumor cells have amplifications and mutations of multiple receptor tyrosine kinases and other downstream signaling kinases. Angiogenesis and immune tolerance are normal physiological processes that are co-opted by the tumor cells for their own growth and proliferation. Therefore, treatment strategies that reverse the co-opted physiological processes, like cytoreduction, radiation, chemotherapy, and TTFields, can potentially provide control of the glioblastoma.

alternating electric fields at frequencies ranging from 100 to 300 kHz disrupt tumor cell cytokinesis during mitosis that results in asymmetric chromosome segregation, aberrant mitotic exit, and immunogenic cell death [27–29]. TTFields monotherapy was compared to chemotherapy for recurrent glioblastoma and the phase III trial showed equivalent efficacy between these two disparate treatment modalities [30]. But patients treated with TTFields experienced fewer adverse events and a better quality of life [30]. Furthermore, the efficacy of TTFields has also been put to test in the newly diagnosed glioblastoma patients. In this chapter, the up-to-date results of the pivotal phase III trial for this population are described.

## Pilot Study of Tumor Treating Fields in Newly Diagnosed Glioblastoma

A pilot study to test the safety of TTFields therapy was conducted from 2005 to 2007 in ten patients with newly diagnosed glioblastoma [31]. The median age of this cohort was 50 (range 32–70) years. All subjects possessed a Karnofsky performance status of 70 or greater and the median Karnofsky was 90. The median overall survival of the cohort was about 56 months and there were two long-term survivors. The first long-term survivor received TTFields and maintenance temozolomide for 12 months, after initial standard radiotherapy and concomitant daily temozolomide. This patient did not develop tumor recurrence and lived for at least another 59 months thereafter [31]. The second long-term survivor was also treated with TTFields and maintenance temozolomide for 12 months, and continued to have no tumor recurrence and lived for an additional 53 months [31]. It is notable that both patients were young, 32 and 33 years respectively, and younger patients are likely to be more responsive to treatment and live longer. In addition, the observed antitumor efficacy supports preclinical data demonstrating an *in vitro* synergistic effect of TTFields with various chemotherapeutic agents in multiple cancer types [32].

## EF-14 was the Second Randomized Trial Using Tumor Treating Fields

This phase III trial enrolled 695 of the planned 700 subjects in a 2:1 ratio between 2009 and 2014, comparing TTFields plus maintenance temozolomide ($n = 466$) with temozolomide alone ($n = 229$) [33]. The primary outcome measure was progression-free survival and secondary endpoints were overall survival, progression-free survival at 6 months, percent 1- and 2-year survival, radiological response based on Macdonald criteria, quality of life assessment (EORTC QLQ-C30) and adverse events severity and frequency [33, 34]. The results of the pre-specified interim analysis have been published, which occurred after 210 subjects were randomized to TTFields plus temozolomide and 105 randomized to temozolomide alone, and was conducted after a median follow-up of 38 (range 18–60) months [35]. Baseline clinical characteristics were balanced and the respective (i) median age was 55 and 57 years, (ii) male:female ratio was 2.0 and 1.8, (iii) corticosteroid use was 24 % and 25 %, (iv) percent completed standard 60 Gy radiotherapy was 91 % and 95 %, and (v) the median number of maintenance temozolomide cycles received was 6 and 4 (Table 8.1) [33, 35]. Both groups had aggressive tumor cytoreduction, and nearly two-thirds of patients underwent gross total resection while another quarter had partial resection [35]. The primary efficacy end-point analysis demonstrated improvement in progression-free survival in the intent-to-treat population of the

**Table 8.1** Baseline patient characteristics and treatment details.

| | All patients (*N*=315) | TTFields plus Temozolomide (*n*=210) | Temozolomide alone (*n*=105) |
|---|---|---|---|
| Age (years) | | | |
| Mean (SD) | 55.8 (11.1) | 55.3 (11.3) | 56.8 (10.5) |
| Median (range) | 57 (20–83) | 57 (20–83) | 58 (21–80) |
| Karnofsky Performance Status score, median (range), %[a] | 90 (60–100) | 90 (60–100) | 90 (70–100) |
| Gender, no. (%) | | | |
| Male | 207 (66) | 140 (67) | 67 (64) |
| Female | 108 (34) | 70 (33) | 38 (36) |
| Use at baseline, no. (%) | | | |
| Antiepileptic medication | 126 (40) | 88 (42) | 38 (36) |
| Corticosteroid therapy | 77 (24) | 51 (24) | 26 (25) |
| Mini-Mental State Examination score, no. (%)[b] | | | |
| ≤26 | 45 (15) | 31 (15) | 14 (13) |
| 27–30 | 247 (78) | 174 (83) | 73 (70) |
| Unknown | 23 (7) | 5 (2) | 18 (17) |
| Extent of resection, no. (%) | | | |
| Biopsy | 34 (11) | 23 (11) | 11 (10) |
| Partial resection | 79 (25) | 52 (25) | 27 (26) |
| Gross total resection | 202 (64) | 135 (64) | 67 (64) |
| Tissue available and tested, no. (%) | 227 (72) | 152 (72) | 75 (71) |
| *MGMT* methylation | 75 (33) | 49 (32) | 26 (35) |
| No methylation | 116 (51) | 79 (52) | 38 (51) |
| Invalid test result | 36 (16) | 24 (16) | 11 (15) |
| Region, no. (%) | | | |
| United States | 191 (61) | 127 (60) | 64 (51) |
| Rest of world | 124 (39) | 83 (40) | 41 (39) |
| Completed radiation therapy, no. (%) <57 Gy | 18 (6) | 13 (6) | 5 (5) |
| 60 Gy (standard ± 5 %) | 291 (92) | 191 (91) | 100 (95) |
| >63 Gy | 6 (2) | 6 (3) | 0 (0) |

(continued)

**Table 8.1** (continued)

| | All patients ($N$=315) | TTFields plus Temozolomide ($n$=210) | Temozolomide alone ($n$=105) |
|---|---|---|---|
| Concomitant temozolomide use, no. (%) | | | |
| Yes | 308 (98) | 207 (99) | 101 (96) |
| Unknown | 7 (2) | 3 (1) | 4 (4) |
| Time from event to randomization, median (range), days | | | |
| Last day of radiotherapy | 37 (13–68) | 36 (13–53) | 38 (13–68) |
| Initial diagnosis | 114 (43–171) | 115 (59–171) | 113 (43–170) |
| No. of maintenance temozolomide cycles until first tumor progression, median (range) | 6 (1–26) | 6 (1–26) | 4 (1–24) |
| Duration of treatment with TTFields, median (range), months | 9 (1–58) | 9 (1–58) | |
| Adherence to TTFields therapy ≥75 % during first 3 months of treatment | | 157 (75) | |

*MGMT* $0^6$-methylguanine-DNA methyltransferase, *TTFields* Tumor Treating Fields
[a]A higher score indicates better functional status
[b]A higher score indicates better cognitive capability

defined interim-analysis dataset and after a median follow-up of 38 months. The median progression-free survival from randomization was 7.1 (95 % CI 5.9–8.2) months in the TTFields plus temozolomide cohort and 4.0 (95 % CI 3.3–5.2) months in the temozolomide alone cohort (hazard ratio=0.62 [95 % CI 0.43–0.89], $p$=0.001) (Fig. 8.2A). In secondary endpoint analyses, the overall survival of the intent-to-treat population showed a median overall survival of 19.6 (95 % CI 16.6–24.4) months in the TTFields plus temozolomide group versus 16.6 (95 % CI 13.6–19.2) months in the temozolomide alone group (hazard ratio=0.74, [95 % CI 0.56–0.98], $p$=0.03) (Fig. 8.2B). The percent of patients alive at 2 years was 43 % and 29 %, respectively ($p$=0.006). When compared to EF-11, the robust efficacy data from EF-14 support the notion that the clinical efficacy of an anti-mitotic treatment, like TTFields, will be more apparent when applied to patients who have undergone aggressive cytoreduction of the tumor, limited use of dexamethasone, and received treatment at an earlier time point of the disease. As patients were allowed to continue the use of TTFields even when tumor recurrence was observed, the data also suggest that extended treatment may still exert an anti-tumor effect even after tumor progression.

Safety and tolerability analysis showed no unexpected grade 3 or 4 adverse events, with nervous system and hematologic events being most common (Table 8.2) [35]. Twenty-two percent of the subjects who received TTFields plus temozolomide ($n$=203) experienced nervous system events, with 7 % seizure and 2 % headache, compared to 25 % who received temozolomide alone ($n$=101), with 8 % seizure and 2 % headache. The respective hematologic disorders were 12 % and 9 %, with 9 % and 3 % thrombocytopenia, 3 % and 1 % neutropenia, 5 % and 5 % leukopenia or lympho-

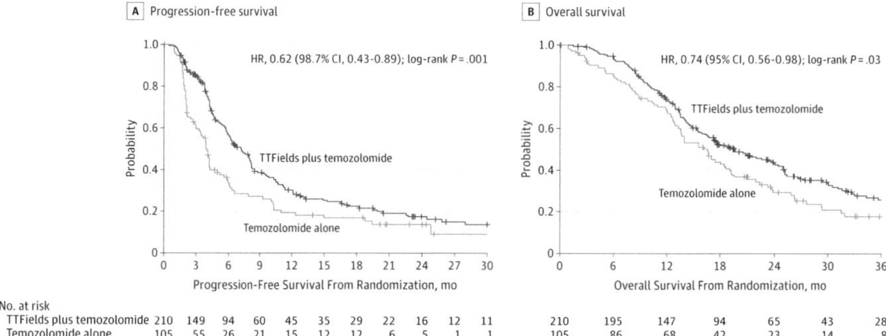


**Fig. 8.2** Survival curves for patients included in the interim analysis in the intent-to-treat population. Survival analyses on time from date of randomization until tumor progression, death, or last follow-up (censored patients) according to the Kaplan-Meier method. (**A**) Progression-free survival and (**B**) overall survival. The *small vertical ticks* on the *curves* indicate censored patients. *HR* hazard ratio, *TTFields* Tumor Treating Fields

**Table 8.2** Grade 3 to 4 treatment-emergent adverse events.

| | No. (%) of Patients With Adverse Events[a] | |
|---|---|---|
| | TTFields Plus Temozolomide (n = 203)[b] | Temozolomide Alone (n = 101)[c] |
| Hematological disorders[d] | 25 (12) | 9 (9) |
| Anemia | 1 (<1) | 2 (2) |
| Leukopenia or lymphopenia | 11 (5) | 5 (5) |
| Neutropenia | 6 (3) | 1 (1) |
| Thrombocytopenia | 19 (9) | 3 (3) |
| Cardiac disorders | 2 (1) | 3 (3) |
| Eye disorders | 2 (1) | 1 (1) |
| Gastrointestinal disorders[d] | 11 (5) | 2 (2) |
| Abdominal pan | 2 (1) | 0 |
| Constipation | 2 (1) | 0 |
| Diarrhea | 1 (<1) | 2 (2) |
| Vomiting | 3 (1) | 1 (1) |
| General disorders | 17 (8) | 5 (5) |
| Fatigue | 8 (4) | 4 (4) |
| Infections | 10 (5) | 5 (5) |
| Injury and procedural complications[d] | 14 (7) | 5 (5) |
| Fall | 6 (3) | 2 (2) |
| Medical device site reaction | 4 (2) | 0 |
| Metabolism and nutrition disorders | 7 (3) | 3 (3) |
| Musculoskeletal disorders | 8 (4) | 3 (3) |
| Nervous system disorders[d] | 45 (22) | 25 (25) |
| Seizure | 15 (7) | 8 (8) |
| Headache | 4 (2) | 2 (2) |

(continued)

**Table 8.2** (continued)

| | No. (%) of Patients With Adverse Events[a] | |
|---|---|---|
| | TTFields Plus Temozolomide (n=203)[b] | Temozolomide Alone (n=101)[c] |
| Psychiatric disorders[d] | 9 (4) | 3 (3) |
| Anxiety | 2 (1) | 0 |
| Bradyphrenia | 0 | 1 (1) |
| Confusional state | 2 (1) | 1 (1) |
| Mental status changes | 4 (2) | 1 (1) |
| Psychotic disorder | 2 (1) | 0 |
| Respiratory disorders | 4 (2) | 1 (1) |
| Skin disorders | 0 | 1 (1) |
| Vascular disorders[d] | 8 (4) | 8 (8) |
| Deep vein thrombosis | 1 (<1) | 3 (3) |
| Pulmonary embolism | 4 (2) | 6 (6) |

*TTFields*, Tumor Treating Fields

[a] Safety is reported on patients who have received any treatment. Randomized patients who never received any maintenance therapy were excluded from this safety analysis

[b] Eight patients died while receiving adjuvant therapy due to causes unrelated to therapy (1 patient for each of the following reasons: cardiac events, pulmonary emboli, respiratory, and infection; and 4 patients with central nervous system disorders likely due to tumor progression)

[c] Four patients died while receiving adjuvant therapy due to causes unrelated to therapy (1 patient for each of the following reasons: cardiac events, pulmonary emboli, respiratory, and unknown)

[d] Patients may have had more than 1 adverse event so subcategories do not total and not all events are subcategorized

penia, and <1 % and 2 % anemia. Site reaction occurred in 2 % of device-treated subjects while 0 % in temozolomide alone subjects, and falls occurred in 3 % and 2 % of the subjects respectively. Therefore, TTFields therapy combined with temozolomide was well-tolerated and exhibited no new side effect from the combination.

## Conclusions

Glioblastoma has significant inter-tumoral and intra-tumoral heterogeneity in molecular characteristics and clinical behavior. Therefore, the prerequisites to demonstrating the clinical efficacy of TTFields are probably related to gross total neurosurgical resection for the purpose of tumor cytoreduction, limited use of immunosuppressive dexamethasone, and intervention at an earlier time point of the disease. Indeed, when TTFields therapy was combined with maintenance temozolomide in the EF-14 phase III trial, the combination was demonstrated to have superiority in both progression-free survival and overall survival when compared to temozolomide alone. Furthermore, the combination was not associated with new or unexpected adverse events. Therefore, the collective data indicate that TTFields treatment, as delivered by the Optune® device, is an important treatment modality for glioblastoma patients.

## References

1. Brennan CW, Verhaak RGW, McKenna A, Campos B, Noushmehr H, Salama SR, et al. The somatic genomic landscape of glioblastoma. Cell. 2013;155:462–77.
2. Verhaak RGW, Hoadley KA, Purdom E, Wang V, Qi Y, Wilkerson MD, et al. Integrated genomic analysis identifies clinically relevant subtypes of glioblastoma characterized by abnormalities in *PDGFRA*, *IDH1*, *EGFR*, and *NF1*. Cancer Cell. 2010;17:98–110.
3. Snuderl M, Fazlollahi L, Le LP, Nitta M, Zhelyazkova BH, Davidson CJ, et al. Mosaic amplification of multiple receptor tyrosine kinase genes in glioblastoma. Cancer Cell. 2011;20:810–7.
4. Sottoriva A, Spiteri I, Piccirillo SGM, Touloumis A, Collins VP, Marioni JC, et al. Intratumor heterogeneity in human glioblastoma reflects cancer evolutionary dynamics. Proc Natl Acad Sci U S A. 2013;110:4009–14.
5. Johnson BE, Mazor T, Hong C, Barnes M, Aihara K, McLean CY, et al. Mutational analysis reveals the origin and therapy-driven evolution of recurrent glioma. Science. 2014;343: 189–93.
6. Wong ET. Tumor growth, invasion, and angiogenesis in malignant gliomas. J Neurooncol. 2006;77:295–6.
7. Romero FJ, Ortega A, Titus F, Ibarra B, Navarro C, Rovira M. Gliomatosis cerebri with formation of a glioblastoma multiforme. Study and follow-up by magnetic resonance and computed tomography. J Comput Tomogr. 1988;12:253–7.
8. Showalter TN, Andrel J, Andrews DW, Curran Jr WJ, Daskalakis C, Werner-Wasik M. Multifocal glioblastoma multiforme: prognostic factors and patterns of progression. Int J Radiat Oncol Biol Phys. 2007;69:820–4.
9. Lun M, Lok E, Gautam S, Wu E, Wong ET. The natural history of extracranial metastasis from glioblastoma multiforme. J Neurooncol. 2011;105:261–73.
10. Müller C, Holtschmidt J, Auer M, Heitzer E, Lamszus E, Schulte A, et al. Hematogenous dissemination of glioblastoma multiforme. Sci Transl Med. 2014;6:247ra101.
11. Chang SM, Wen P, Cloughesy T, Greenberg H, Schiff D, Conrad C, et al. Phase II study of CCI-779 in patients with recurrent glioblastoma multiforme. Invest New Drugs. 2005;23:357–61.
12. Lee EQ, Kaley TJ, Duda DG, Schiff D, Lassman AB, Wong ET, et al. A multicenter, phase II, randomized, noncomparative clinical trial of radiation and temozolomide with or without vandetanib in newly diagnosed glioblastoma patients. Clin Cancer Res. 2015;21:3610–8.
13. Jain RK. Normalization of tumor vasculature: an emerging concept in antiangiogenic therapy. Science. 2005;307:58–62.
14. Gilbert MR, Dignam JJ, Armstrong TS, Wefel JS, Blumenthal DT, et al. A randomized trial of bevacizumab for newly diagnosed glioblastoma. N Engl J Med. 2014;370:699–708.
15. Chinot OL, Wick W, Mason W, Henriksson R, Saran F, Nishkawa R, et al. Bevacizumab plus radiotherapy-temozolomide for newly diagnosed glioblastoma. N Engl J Med. 2014;370:709–22.
16. Parsa AT, Waldron JS, Panner A, Crane CA, Parney IF, Barry JJ, et al. Loss of tumor suppressor PTEN function increases B7-H1 expression and immunoresistance in glioma. Nat Med. 2006;13:84–8.
17. Bloch O, Crane CA, Kaur R, Safaee M, Rutkowski MJ, Parsa AT. Gliomas promote immunosuppression through induction of B7-H1 expression in tumor-associated macrophages. Clin Cancer Res. 2013;19:3165–75.
18. Wong ET, Lok E, Gautam S, Swanson KD. Dexamethasone exerts profound immunologic interference on treatment efficacy for recurrent glioblastoma. Br J Cancer. 2015;113:232–41.
19. Hughes MA, Parisi M, Grossman SA, Kleinberg L. Primary brain tumors treated with steroids and radiotherapy: low CD4 counts and risk of infection. Int J Radiat Oncol Biol Phys. 2005;62:1423–6.

20. Pitter KL, Tamagno I, Alikhanyan K, Hosni-Ahmed A, Pattwell SS, Donnola S, et al. Corticosteroids compromise survival in glioblastoma. Brain. 2016;139:1458–71.
21. Grossman SA, Ye X, Lesser G, Sloan A, Carraway H, Desideri S, et al. Immunosuppression in patients with high-grade gliomas treated with radiation and temozolomide. Clin Cancer Res. 2011;17:5473–80.
22. Back MF, Ang EL, Ng WH, See SJ, Lim CC, Chan SP, et al. Improved median survival for glioblastoma multiforme following introduction of adjuvant temozolomide chemotherapy. Ann Acad Med Singapore. 2007;36:338–42.
23. Takano S, Kimu H, Tsuda K, Osuka S, Nakai K, Yamamoto T, et al. Decrease in the apparent diffusion coefficient in peritumoral edema for the assessment of recurrent glioblastoma treated by bevacizumab. Acta Neurochir Suppl. 2013;118:185–9.
24. Chu K, Jeong SW, Jung KH, Han SY, Lee ST, Kim M, et al. Celecoxib induces functional recovery after intracerebral hemorrhage with reduction of brain edema and perihematomal cell death. J Cereb Blood Flow Metab. 2004;24:926–33.
25. Lee SH, Park HK, Ryu WS, Lee JS, Bae HJ, Han MK, et al. Effects of celecoxib on hematoma and edema volumes in primary intracerebral hemorrhage: a multicenter randomized controlled trial. Eur J Neurol. 2013;20:1161–9.
26. Carpentier AF, Ferrari D, Bailon O, Ursu R, Banissi C, Dubessy AL, et al. Steroid-sparing effects of angiotensin-II inhibitors in glioblastoma patients. Eur J Neurol. 2012;19:1337–42.
27. Kirson ED, Gurvich Z, Schneiderman R, Dekel E, Itzhaki A, Wasserman Y, et al. Disruption of cancer cell replication by alternating electric fields. Cancer Res. 2004;64:3288–95.
28. Gera N, Yang A, Holtzman TS, Lee SX, Wong ET, Swanson KD. Tumor treating fields perturb the localization of septins and cause aberrant mitotic exit. PLoS One. 2015;10:e0125269.
29. Lee SX, Wong E, Swanson K. Disruption of cell division within anaphase by tumor treating electric fields (TTFields) leads to immunogenic cell death. Neuro-Oncology. 2013;15 Suppl 3:iii66–7.
30. Stupp R, Wong ET, Kanner AA, Steinberg D, Engelhard H, Heidecke V, et al. NovoTTF-100A versus physician's choice chemotherapy in recurrent glioblastoma: a randomized phase III trial of a novel treatment modality. Eur J Cancer. 2012;48:2192–202.
31. Rulseh AM, Keller J, Klener J, Sroubek J, Dbalý V, Syrucek M, et al. Long-term survival of patients suffering from glioblastoma multiforme treated with tumor-treating fields. World J Surg Oncol. 2012;10:220.
32. Kirson ED, Schneiderman RS, Dbalý V, Tovaryš F, Vymazal J, Itzhaki A, et al. Chemotherapeutic treatment efficacy and sensitivity are increased by adjuvant alternating electric fields (TTFields). BMC Med Phys. 2009;9:1.
33. https://clinicaltrials.gov/ct2/show/NCT00916409.
34. Macdonald DR, Casino TL, Schold Jr SC, Cairncross JG. Response criteria for phase II studies of supratentorial malignant glioma. J Clin Oncol. 1990;8:1277–80.
35. Stupp R, Taillibert S, Kanner AA, Kesari S, Steinberg DM, Toms SA, et al. Maintenance therapy with tumor-treating fields plus temozolomide vs temozolomide alone for glioblastoma. A randomized clinical trial. JAMA. 2015;314:2535–43.

# Chapter 9
# Supportive Care in Patients Using Tumor Treating Fields Therapy

**Mario E. Lacouture, John DeNigris, and Andrew A. Kanner**

Optune® is a cancer treatment device that uses alternating electric fields or Tumor Treating Fields (TTFields) to provide local therapy for a patient's tumor. It has received approval for two indications from the U.S. Food and Drug Administration, the first in 2011 for recurrent glioblastoma and the second in 2015 for newly diagnosed glioblastoma. The initial approval in patients with recurrent glioblastoma was based on the device's (i) comparable treatment efficacy when compared to systemic chemotherapy, (ii) absence of serious adverse events, and (iii) improved quality of life (QoL) [1, 2]. Furthermore, no new or unexpected adverse events were noted in the post-approval patient registry [3]. The second approval resulted from favorable progression-free survival and overall survival in the device-treatment arm in combination with maintenance temozolomide after a pre-specified interim analysis [4]. There was also no unexpected adverse event and the QoL outcome appeared to be similar in both arms. However, dermatologic adverse events (dAEs) remain an important issue among patients receiving TTFields therapy. In this chapter, the prevention, diagnosis, and management of dAEs are discussed in the first section while the QoL analyses from both pivotal phase III clinical trials are reviewed in the second section.

M.E. Lacouture (✉)
Oncodermatology Service, Memorial Sloan Kettering Cancer Center, New York, NY, USA
e-mail: LacoutuM@mskcc.org

J. DeNigris
Morsani College of Medicine, University of South Florida, Tampa, FL, USA

A.A. Kanner, M.D. (✉)
Stereotactic Radiosurgery Unit, Department of Neurosurgery, Tel Aviv Sourasky Medical Center, Tel Aviv University, Tel Aviv, Israel
e-mail: andrewk@tlvmc.gov.il



E.T. Wong (ed.), *Alternating Electric Fields Therapy in Oncology*,
DOI 10.1007/978-3-319-30576-9_9

## Dermatologic Adverse Events Associated with Tumor Treating Fields Therapy

TTFields are delivered by ceramic discs located on two pairs of transducer arrays. These discs have a layer of hydrogel to ensure conductive contact with the scalp and they are adherent to the patient's shaved head by hypoallergenic medical tape. While systemic adverse events have not been reported, the continuous application of the transducer arrays results in a new category of dAEs, with contact dermatitis and skin infections being the most prominent ones [2]. Knowledge of the mechanisms by which these dAEs develop, as well as strategies for prevention and treatment are critical to maintain QoL and consistency of device utilization.

### *Pathophysiology of Dermatologic Adverse Events*

The epidermis is composed of keratinocytes, melanocytes, Langerhans cells, and Merkel cells. The doubling time of human keratinocytes is every 24 hours, with transit time from the basal layer to the stratum corneum taking at least 14 days. Further transit from the stratum corneum to desquamation requires an additional 14 days [5] and therefore a complete turnover of the epidermis takes a total of 28 days. Cells from the innate arm of the immune system, including macrophages, antigen-presenting cells, and natural killer cells reside in the epidermis. When there is an insult to the skin, lymphocytes from the adaptive immune system may temporarily take residence in the epidermis. These immune cells are responsible for the observed contact dermatitis that may develop upon exposure to some of the components of the Optune® device.

Transducer arrays are directly applied to the scalp for at least 18 hours a day and left in place for 3 to 4 days at a time. During an array exchange, the previous ones are removed and new ones are placed on the scalp in a slightly relocated fashion to reduce prolonged direct contact. Distinctive mechanical, thermal, chemical, and moisture-related stresses occur if the arrays are applied repeatedly to the same area of the skin. Given the potential for causing dAEs, meticulous monitoring of the skin condition and timely exchange of the arrays are highly recommended.

Hair directly affects the quality of array-to-scalp contact. There are approximately 100,000 hair follicles on the scalp, and around 100 shafts of hair shed each day [6]. An outward pressure to the adhered transducers arrays is generated by a growth rate of 0.2 to 0.5 mm per day. To minimize the effect of this pressure, the scalp should be shaved every time when the arrays are exchanged.

Surgery will invariably result in the formation of a scar on the incised skin. Scars arise due to fibrous tissue proliferation during the replacement of previously normal skin where integrity is compromised. Although a scar continues to remodel for up to 1 year after surgical incision, the skin on the scar does not fully regain its original mechanical strength. It is estimated that scars have only 70 % of the tensile strength of normal skin [7]. Moreover, altered circulation through scar tissue increases patient susceptibility to dAEs when ceramic discs are placed immediately over them [7].

Abnormal stimuli to the skin are the catalysts that produce pathological changes. TTFields therapy potentially exposes skin to stimuli such as repetitive mechanical trauma, resulting in inflammation, infection, and wound healing complications at the site of previous surgical scars. The shaved scalp that was previously covered by hair may be exposed to ambient ultraviolet radiation and this may result in inflammatory changes [7]. Multiple risk factors have been found to increase the risk of developing dAEs. The first would include placing the ceramic discs from the arrays directly over scars or craniotomy hardware. Another risk factor occurs in patients who have previously developed a contact dermatitis reaction to any materials that are in the arrays. Those with hyperhidrosis (excessive sweating) have been found to have a higher complication rate due to the hydrophilic nature of hydrogel, which may liquefy at high ambient temperature and upon exposure to sweat. Additionally, there is an increased risk for individuals with a history of skin exposure to radiation, either ultraviolet and/or ionizing radiation, and those who are also being treated with systemic anti-cancer agents, high doses of corticosteroid, or both [7].

## *Specific Dermatologic Pathologies*

Five types of potential pathologies leading to dAEs have been noted with the use of TTFields therapy (Table 9.1), including (i) allergic contact dermatitis (ACD), (ii) irritant contact dermatitis (ICD), (iii) erosions, (iv) ulcers, and (v) skin infections or pustules [7]. These processes may occur independently or coexist at sites where the scalp makes contact with the arrays. Chemical irritation from the hydrogel, moisture and/or alcohol may directly lead to ICD, while allergy to the adhesive tape and/or hydrogel may cause a delayed form of ACD. Erosions from mechanical trauma may occur from shaving, array application, or array removal. Ischemic injury produced by pressure from the arrays may lead to ulcer formation. Ultimately, infection with or without pustules may occur when the skin is affected by pathogenic bacteria [7].

ACD and ICD are the two types of inflammation that patients may develop when using TTFields therapy [7]. ACD is characterized by an inflammatory reaction to specific exogenous allergens that come into contact with the skin. In this case, an individual must become sensitized to the allergen [8]. Resolution of ACD not only requires removing the allergen, but may also necessitate the use of topical corticosteroids to quell the inflammatory reaction. In contrast, ICD is a nonspecific type of inflammation caused by direct cell damage upon contact with a substance that is inherently harmful to cells [8]. Removal of the irritant is sufficient and the inflammation will resolve with time.

Erosions are characteristically described as delineated, moist, and depressed lesions resulting from disruption of a part or all of the epidermis [7]. Mild bleeding with pain or burning may also be present [9]. These changes may occur after trauma from the arrays, shaving injury, inflammation or maceration due to sweat, rupture of

**Table 9.1** Potential causes of dermatologic adverse events (dAEs)

| Adverse events | Potential cause | Intervention |
|---|---|---|
| Contact dermatitis | Allergy | Topical steroid |
| | • Tape | • Clobetasol |
| | • Hydrogel | • Betamethasone |
| | Chemical irritation | Array placement |
| | • Hydrogel | |
| | • Moisture (sweat) | |
| | • Alcohol | |
| Erosion and ulcers | Mechanical trauma | Array placement |
| | • Shaving | |
| | • Array pressure/removal | Topical antibiotics |
| | | • Mupriocin |
| | Array pressure leading to decreased perfusion | • Clindamycin |
| Skin infections and pustules | Secondary bacterial infection | Topical or oral antibiotics |
| | | • Cefadroxil |
| | | • Mupriocin |
| | | • Clindamycin |

vesicles or bullae from infection, as well as epidermal necrosis. Typically, erosions do not result in scarring [7].

Ulcers represent a more severe form of dAEs in which loss of the epidermis and dermis has occurred, and therefore increasing the risk of scarring [7]. Ulcers may be necrotic or clean, and during the healing process may contain granulation tissue. As the ulcer heals, dried blood, serum, and exudate may form a crust [7]. Infection of the ulcerated skin is indicated by purulent, granular, or malodorous discharge.

With the abundance of microbes that exist on the skin, infection is common [10]. Pustules represent a purulent infection in the epidermis composed of leukocytes, cellular debris (yellow color), and bacteria (greenish-yellow color) [7]. White pus may represent sterile inflammatory reaction without the presence of microorganisms. Vesicles and bullae are fluid-filled lesions with clear content that may or may not be infected. They may arise from early viral infections or trauma by friction or shearing forces. When bullae are due to bacterial infection, they are called bullous impetigo [7].

## *Management of Dermatologic Adverse Events*

Adverse events on the skin associated with TTFields therapy can be prophylactically prevented and intervened with specific treatments depending on the type of dAE. Prevention is preferred, but prompt recognition of dAEs is also important. Early signs that a dAE is developing may include erythema, edema, scaling, discharge, crusting, pain, pruritis, erosions, or any of the above in combination [7].

Prophylaxis is an important preventive measure that will preclude or limit adverse events on the skin. First and foremost, both patient and caregiver should be educated to recognize potential dAEs and, because they are the individuals preparing the scalp and exchanging the arrays, it is critical that they should have intimate knowledge about the skin integrity as well as appropriate training to apply and remove the arrays. The treating oncologist should also be available to manage these adverse events when they develop to ensure timely intervention.

Scalp preparation, if done correctly, will lower the risk of irritating the skin and also optimize the delivery of TTFields. Conditions on the scalp that can contribute to dAEs include hair length, moisture from sweat, existence of sebum, and the length of time the same set of arrays contact the skin. Modification of these conditions can lower the risk of dAEs. Access to the scalp requires removing arrays and thus proper scalp preparation is essential at each subsequent replacement of arrays.

Proper and timely shaving using an electric razor is recommended to maximize the closeness of the shave and to ensure array contact on the scalp. All effort to avoid cutting the skin should be taken and therefore a straight blade razor is not recommended. Once the skin has been compromised there is a concomitant increased risk of developing dAEs. To test the closeness of the shave, one can use gauze or a cotton ball soaked with 70 % isopropyl alcohol and run it across the scalp. Detectable friction or resistance would indicate the need for a closer shave [7]. Furthermore, mineral oil should be applied before shaving because it allows for cleansing of the skin and facilitates the removal of bacteria and scale.

In order to adequately remove sebum from the scalp, fragrance-free shampoo should be used after shaving. Once rinsed, the scalp should be wiped with 70 % isopropyl alcohol. By eliminating as much sebum as possible, the contact between arrays and scalp is enhanced.

Although each transducer array is stored in sterilized individual packages, other precautions to prevent infection are required. Prior to any exchange of the arrays, proper hand washing, sanitizing the electric razor, and cleaning of the scalp are recommended [7]. The use of 70 % isopropyl alcohol will help sterilize the skin surface. In addition, the patient's electric razor should not be shared with other individuals.

Transducer array application and removal is a critical step in preventing dAEs. The layout takes into account the head size, tumor size, and tumor location in the patient. Although each array is placed according to the layout plan, avoiding sites of surgical scars and craniotomy closure hardware is important when placing the arrays. Skin breakdown, erosions, ulcerations, or any combination of dAEs may occur if the ceramic discs are applied over scars or hardware. The concurrent administration of anti-cancer agents such as temozolomide or bevacizumab may also impair normal skin turnover and wound healing, increasing the possibility of erosions or ulcerations.

During array re-application, which occurs approximately every 3 to 4 days, the position should be shifted approximately 0.75 inch (or 20 mm) from the prior location. In doing so, the hydrogel layer is re-positioned to an area between the prior contact sites [7]. Indentation of the surface of the scalp will indicate the last location of the ceramic discs. Due to individual patient factors such as hyperhidrosis, some patients may require more frequent array changes. Less skin irritation will occur when arrays are removed carefully and without excessive force. Slow and even tension is recommended during removal, which takes approximately 60 seconds per array. If the arrays become difficult to remove, mineral oil can be applied directly to the scalp at the edges of the arrays to facilitate removal and to minimize the need to use excessive force. To avoid irritating the scalp, rubbing the skin to remove the remaining adhesives should be avoided and mineral oil should be applied to help dissolve the adhesive.

Patients and caregivers must be educated on proper scalp care during TTFields treatment. The hydrogel associated with the ceramic discs is hydrophilic, and may partially liquefy after physical activity or warmer weather due to increased sweating. Under these circumstances, changing the arrays on a more frequent basis, such as once every 1 to 2 days, may be necessary [7]. The risk of negative skin reactions and poor wound healing may increase when systemic medications are combined with TTFields therapy (see below). Likely culprits include prolonged use of corticosteroids, systemic chemotherapies, and targeted anti-cancer drugs.

Treatment interventions should be considered after a patient has developed dAEs. As defined by preclinical studies, the electric field frequency and intensity therapeutic parameters are preset into the device and cannot be modified. Therefore, this creates a predetermined "dose" that cannot be changed by the treating oncologist [7]. However, dAEs may be treated by pharmacological intervention, treatment interruption, or both. As discussed previously as a means of prophylactic intervention, relocating the arrays and avoiding the affected skin can also be used for treatment of established dAEs. For areas that cannot be avoided by simply shifting the arrays, sterile nonadherent dressing pads or gauzes can be inserted between ceramic discs and scalp surfaces with dAEs to temporarily avoid direct contact.

Pharmacological treatment primarily consists of topical therapies, such as corticosteroids and antibiotics. Dermatitis is primarily treated with topical corticosteroids. Since topical therapies can only be applied at the time of transducer array exchange, high-potency corticosteroid ointments or foams are recommended. When the epidermal barrier is compromised or signs of infection exist, topical antibiotics should be used. Skin flora on the scalp should designate the selected spectrum of antibiotics used. However, neomycin containing topical antibiotics should be avoided due to a high incidence of ACD in the general population.

Topical therapies should be applied and left for 15 to 30 minutes. Residue must be removed by either re-washing the scalp or by using 70 % isopropyl alcohol. Lipids in the creams and ointments may interfere with contact of the ceramic discs in the transducer arrays when residue remains on the skin. An alternative is the use of topical steroids and antibiotics that are delivered in a vehicle such as foam, which will dissolve within minutes after skin contact.

Treatment interruption and topical therapies may be required for patients suffering from intolerable dAEs. Discontinued array application for 2 to 7 days is frequently sufficient for the resolution of the dAEs in concordance with the cellular turnover rate in the epidermis [7]. However, the treating oncologist should recognize that prolonged treatment interruption may compromise TTFields therapy efficacy as longer survival was noted among patients who had a compliance rate of ≥75 % when compared to those with <75 % compliance [3]. Given the likelihood of recurrence in glioblastoma patients, prophylactic measures to prevent dAEs are particularly important and should be used upon TTFields therapy re-application.

## *Dermatologic Adverse Events Associated with Combination Therapies*

As TTFields therapy is approved for the treatment of glioblastoma, most patients have undergone or are still undergoing other forms of therapy. Frequently, patients will have healing scars from previous surgery. They may also be receiving concomitant systemic chemotherapy. Both situations complicate the use of transducer arrays, and should prompt the oncologist to monitor more frequent for severe dAEs. As each systemic chemotherapy or targeted drug therapy has its own unique adverse event profile, only treatments that are commonly used together with TTFields therapy will be discussed (Table 9.2).

Bevacizumab has been found to delay wound healing, including surgical wound closure [11, 12]. By inhibiting the vascular endothelial growth factor ligand, bevacizumab blocks angiogenesis, which is required for proper wound healing. Furthermore, the repetition of applying and removing transducer arrays, as well as shaving of the hair, from the scalp can expose the skin to frequent mechanical

**Table 9.2** Preventive measures for TTFields combination therapy

| Treatment | Mechanism of contribution to adverse event | Precautionary measures |
|---|---|---|
| Bevacizumab | Delayed wound healing | • Avoid placing arrays at sites of surgical scars, recent surgical sites, sites of erosions/ulcerations<br>• During manipulation of skin, take extra care to avoid compromising the skin barrier |
| Craniotomy | Inferior tensile strength of skin | • Avoid placing arrays at sites of surgical scars, recent surgical sites |
| | Altered vascular supply to skin | |
| Temozolomide | Myelosuppression | • Close monitoring for secondary infections<br>• Close monitoring for bleeding<br>• Close monitoring for rashes |
| Radiation | Radiation-induced cell death | • Careful manipulation of skin at sites of radiation exposure |

trauma [13, 14]. These factors combined with delayed wound healing will likely increase the frequency and severity of dAEs. Therefore, array placement at areas with compromised skin, such as previous surgical sites, must be avoided. When dAEs are detected, arrays must be placed in alternative areas. Furthermore, the oncologist caring for patients who are receiving concurrent bevacizumab needs to be aware of compromised wound healing, and extra care must be taken when manipulating their skin. Extra effort will also be needed to ensure proper prophylactic intervention in these patients to prevent significant morbidities associated with improper wound healing [15].

Temozolomide is a cytotoxic agent for glioblastoma patients and it has been found to cause neutropenia and thrombocytopenia [16]. If damage to the skin occurs during preparation or manipulation of the device, neutropenic or thrombocytopenic patients would be at a higher risk of developing secondary infections or severe bleeding, respectively. In addition, rashes have been reported in up to 4 % of patient's receiving temozolomide [17]. Monitoring these potential adverse events is critical given the increased susceptibility of these patients when using TTFields therapy concurrently. Although no studies to date have linked temozolomide to complications with wound healing, cell death induced by DNA alkylation [18] could potentially interfere with this process.

Radiation commonly compromises wound healing and can lead to atrophy of the skin, ulcer formation, and desquamation [19]. Up to 60 % of surgical patients who were previously treated with radiation experience complications [19]. Increased rates of infection and poor wound healing have been reported [16], likely resulting from death of skin cells and infiltration of immune cells at the site of radiation exposure. Patients with glioblastoma are typically treated with radiation to the head, leading to an increased likelihood of dAEs on the scalp when transducer arrays are applied. One must account for the repetitive mechanical forces that will be applied to the fragile, irradiated skin and adjust accordingly.

The initial recommended treatment of glioblastoma is surgical resection [20]. Thus, craniotomy scars will be present in the majority of patients. Scars that have not completely healed have inferior tensile strength and altered blood flow [11], and therefore they are more susceptible to developing dAEs. It is important to allow all scars to heal completely before array placement, and to refrain from placing arrays directly over these areas. In addition, proper post-operative wound care to surgical sites is highly recommended.

Patients with glioblastoma may also be treated with various combinations of anti-cancer therapies. As most patients will have undergone a craniotomy, treatment with bevacizumab in patients with craniotomy scars is common. Patients who have undergone a craniotomy and who are concomitantly treated with bevacizumab have been shown to have higher rates of wound healing complications post-operatively [15]. Therefore, with the application of transducer arrays and the use of TTFields therapy, applying proper prophylactic therapies and monitoring for dAEs are critical for these patients.

## *Conclusion*

TTFields therapy is a novel anti-cancer treatment that involves physical contact of the transducer arrays with the scalp and has a unique profile of adverse events. The treating oncologist and other staff members must become familiar with these adverse events, and develop individualized plans for preventing and treating them. The continuous use of proper prophylactic measures, combined with the necessary treatment interventions when adverse events develop, are essential in managing patients on TTFields therapy. Moreover, the concurrent use of systemic agents, surgery or radiation may potentiate the frequency and severity of dAEs, requiring additional supportive care efforts, all of which will help to maintain QoL and maximize benefit from TTFields.

## Quality of Life Issues in Patients Treated with Tumor Treating Fields Therapy

Tumor control and survival had traditionally been the primary focus of brain tumor treatment assessment. Clinical research was designed around clinical outcome parameters, which included primarily overall and progression-free survival as endpoints. The emphasis was on extending life and less so on QoL. Although the concept of QoL in this context has been recognized for a long time, there has been a clear shift to more QoL-oriented medicine over the last 2 to 3 decades [21]. Functional performance has become another important assessment parameter of cancer patients after Karnofsky introduced a simple performance score, but an appreciation of its importance on survival and treatment response has led to a shift in what is considered therapeutic success in cancer clinical trials [22].

The assessment of QoL has therefore evolved into an important and fundamental part of oncologic trials as well as part of the routine protocol at clinical follow-up visits. QoL assessment consists of a number of domains that cover a multitude of aspects of performance and well-being, and tries to reflect the current social, economic, psychological, spiritual, and health status of the individual patient. Organ-specific QoL questionnaires for cancer patients have been designed and validated in order to characterize the disease-specific impact on an individual's life [23, 24]. In brain tumor patients—more than in other cancer patients—the disease affects multiple domains of well-being and performance. Patients often suffer from a multitude of neurological deficiencies and symptoms, seizures, and side effects from high-dose corticosteroids and anticonvulsive therapies, even before the initiation of prolonged radiation and chemotherapy [25].

The purpose of this section of the chapter is to summarize QoL issues related to the usage of TTFields therapy in patients with glioblastoma, a World Health Organization grade IV primary brain tumor and the most common primary malignant brain tumor affecting the adult population.

## *Quality of Life Assessment During Tumor Treating Fields Therapy*

In contrast to conventional chemotherapies, biological therapies, and radiation treatment, TTFields therapy involves an externally applied device whose technical details [2, 4] and proposed mechanism of function have been described in depth elsewhere [26, 27]. Relevant for this review is the fact that continued treatment is applied through transducer arrays that are attached to the shaved scalp. These arrays are connected to a portable device that generates TTFields and, as such, affects tumor growth. This is the source of the main difference between its application to traditional drug treatments, and the reason why it might impact QoL in a different way. Scalp attached transducer arrays are connected and activated by the operating device for at least 18 hours a day in order to deliver effective treatment. As a result, patients and their families become closely involved in the provision of treatment and can take responsibility for its correct application on a daily basis.

Two phase III randomized clinical trials involving the application of the device in glioblastoma patients have thus far been conducted. The first trial (EF-11) compared TTFields monotherapy to Best Physician's Choice chemotherapy in glioblastoma patients with one or more recurrences. This trial included 120 patients randomized to the device arm, and the results were published elsewhere [2]. The second trial (EF-14) compared temozolomide maintenance therapy with and without TTFields therapy in over 700 newly diagnosed glioblastoma patients after completion of initial standard-of-care radiotherapy and concomitant daily temozolomide in multiple treatment centers. The results of the interim analysis on 315 analyzed patients were recently published [4] and the QoL-related results of both clinical trials are discussed here.

## *Outcome of Quality of Life Assessment*

One of the important questions related to the use of the device in real life is patient compliance. The log file analyses that were generated by the device of patients treated in the EF-11 trial revealed a high mean compliance rate (86 %, range 41–98 %) that translated into a mean use of 20.6 hours per day. Completion of at least 1 month of treatment (i.e., a 4-week cycle) was documented in 79 out of 120 (65.8 %) enrolled patients in the TTFields therapy arm. A *post hoc* subgroup analysis showed a trend towards better compliance and treatment efficacy [28].

There are no known systemic adverse events associated with the Optune® device, except for an occasional skin rash, itching, irritation or, in rare cases, skin ulceration. These adverse events are associated with the use of the scalp transducer arrays and defined as mild-to-moderate (grade 1 or 2) contact dermatitis, occurring in 16 % of patients [2]. The dermatologic aspects of this therapeutic approach were presented in detail and discussed in the early part of this chapter.

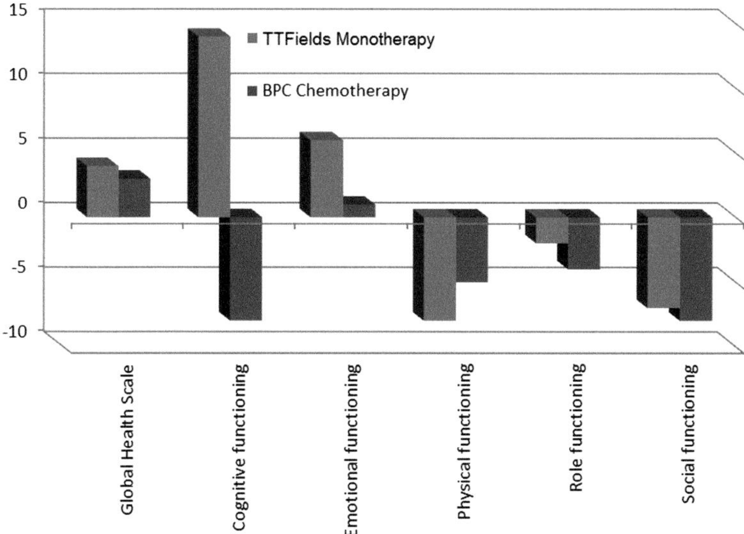


**Fig. 9.1** Longitudinal change in QoL domains as recorded on the QLQ C-30 questionnaire from baseline to 3 months in the EF-11 trial. Change in % from baseline (negative values suggest worsening of the domain). *BPC* Best Physician's Choice, *QLQ* quality of life questionnaire, *QoL* quality of life

Participating patients in the EF-11 trial answered a standard QoL questionnaire (EORTC-QLQ C-30) [29] at the time of enrollment and every 3 months thereafter. A total of 63 (26 %) of those patients were available for a longitudinal QoL analysis (>3 months on study). Thirty-nine out of 120 (30 %) patients treated with TTFields monotherapy and 27 out of 117 (23 %) who received chemotherapy were eligible for a longitudinal QoL analysis. The QoL domains comprised a global health scale, as well as cognitive, emotional, physical, role and social functioning (Fig. 9.1). A striking difference was observed between the chemotherapy arm and the TTFields monotherapy arm in the domains of cognitive and emotional functioning, favoring the latter. There were no remarkable differences in global health, social, role, or physical functioning between the two treatment arms. In addition, treatment-associated toxicity was assessed by a symptom scale analysis (Fig. 9.2). As expected, appetite loss, constipation, diarrhea, nausea, and vomiting were predominantly associated with patients in the chemotherapy-treated arm. Pain and fatigue were reported only by patients in the chemotherapy arm and none in the TTFields-treated group.

The results of the EF-14 trial have only been published partially. The following are data of the interim analysis, after the completion of data collection on the first 315 randomized patients [4]. A total of 238 (75.6 %) patients who were enrolled in EF-14 were available for this longitudinal QoL analysis (>3 months into the study). Within this group, 171 out of 210 (81.4 %) received combined TTFields therapy and temozolomide and 67 out of 105 (63.8 %) treated with temozolomide only were eligible for this interim analysis. It should be borne in mind that both arms received standard temozolomide chemotherapy and that the study arm was additionally

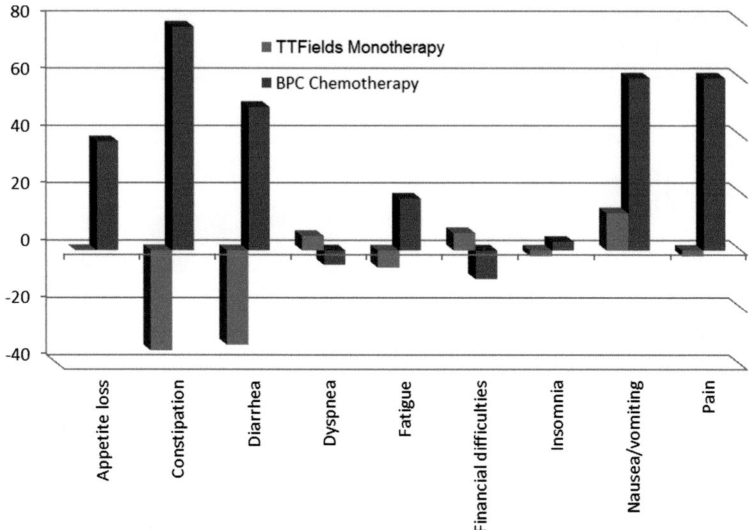


**Fig. 9.2** Longitudinal change in symptom scale from baseline to 3 months in the EF-11 trial as recorded by a questionnaire. Change in % from baseline (negative values suggest improvement of symptoms). *BPC* Best Physician's Choice

treated with TTFields therapy. Chemotherapy-associated symptoms were more evenly distributed between the two study arms. In EF-14, the QoL domains were similar over a 9- to 12-month longitudinal observation period. A statistical analysis (two-way ANOVA) did not yield any meaningful differences yet.

## Conclusions

Glioblastoma patients may have a number of treatment options at certain stages of their disease, and while the effectiveness of the various approaches might be quite similar, the therapeutic approach that has a superior QoL profile will be more appealing for the patient. As a result, a substantial portion of current cancer clinical trials is devoted to QoL issues. Patients with recurrent glioblastoma treated with TTFields monotherapy reported more favorable QoL outcomes and fewer adverse events compared to patients who were in the chemotherapy group in the EF-11 trial. However, in EF-14, chemotherapy-associated symptoms were more evenly distributed between the two study arms; the QoL domains were similar over a 9- to 12-month longitudinal observation period and there was no significant difference in any of the QoL domains. Taken together, TTFields monotherapy showed a more favorable QoL profile compared to chemotherapy alone, while TTFields in combination with chemotherapy did not impact the QoL of patients compared to chemotherapy alone.

**Acknowledgement** The author is very grateful to Esther Eshkol for editorial assistance in the preparation of this manuscript and to Tal Shahar, MD and Uri Rozovski, MD for aiding with the quality of life statistical analysis.

## References

1. http://www.fda.gov/NewsEvents/Newsroom/PressAnnouncements/ucm251669.htm.
2. Stupp R, Wong ET, Kanner AA, Steinberg D, Engelhard H, Heidecke V, et al. NovoTTF-100A versus physician's choice chemotherapy in recurrent glioblastoma: a randomised phase III trial of a novel treatment modality. Eur J Cancer. 2012;48(14):2192–202.
3. Mrugala MM, Engelhard HH, Tran D, Kew Y, Cavaliere R, Villano JL, et al. Clinical practice experience with NovoTTF-100A™ system for glioblastoma: The Patient Registry Dataset (PRiDe). Semin Oncol. 2014;41 Suppl 6:S4–13.
4. Stupp R, Taillibert S, Kanner AA, Kesari S, Steinberg DM, Toms SA, et al. Maintenance therapy with tumor-treating fields plus temozolomide vs temozolomide alone for glioblastoma. A randomized clinical trial. JAMA. 2015;314:2535–43.
5. Rheinwald JG, Green H. Epidermal growth factor and the multiplication of cultured human epidermal keratinocytes. Nature. 1977;265(5593):421–4.
6. Stenn KS, Paus R. Controls of hair follicle cycling. Physiol Rev. 2001;81(1):449–94.
7. Lacouture ME, Davids ME, Elzinga G, Butowski N, Tran D, Villano J, et al. Characterization and management of dermatologic adverse events with the NovoTTF-100A System, a novel anti-mitotic electric field device for the treatment of recurrent glioblastoma. Semin Oncol. 2014;41 Suppl 4:S1–14.
8. Bourke J, Coulson I, English J. Guidelines for the management of contact dermatitis: an update. Br J Dermatol. 2009;160(5):946–54.
9. Malak JA, Kibbi AG. Revised terminology in dermatology: a call for the new millennium. Arch Dermatol. 2001;137(1):93–4.
10. Grice EA, Segre JA. The skin microbiome: our second genome. Annu Rev Genomics Hum Genet. 2012;13:151–70.
11. Hardy MA. The biology of scar formation. Phys Ther. 1989;69(12):1014–24.
12. Chen HX, Cleck JN. Adverse effects of anticancer agents that target the VEGF pathway. Nat Rev Clin Oncol. 2009;6(8):465–77.
13. Cruickshank CN. The microanatomy of the epidermis in relation to trauma. J Tissue Viability. 2006;16(2):16–9.
14. Cowley K, Vanoosthuyze K. Insights into shaving and its impact on skin. Br J Dermatol. 2012;166 Suppl 1:6–12.
15. Ladha H, Pawar T, Gilbert MR, Mandel J, O'Brien B, Conrad C, et al. Wound healing complications in brain tumor patients on bevacizumab. J Neurooncol. 2015;124(3):501–6.
16. Stupp R, Hegi ME, Mason WP, van den Bent MJ, Taphoorn MJ, Janzer RC, et al. Effect of radiotherapy with concomitant and adjuvant temozolomide versus radiotherapy alone on survival in glioblastoma in a randomized phase III study: 5-year analysis of the EORTC-NCIC trial. Lancet Oncol. 2009;10(5):459–66.
17. Brada M, Hoang-Xuan K, Rampling R, Dietrich PY, Dirix LY, Macdonald D, et al. Multicenter phase II trial of temozolomide in patients with glioblastoma multiforme at first relapse. Ann Oncol. 2001;12(2):259–66.
18. Agarwala SS, Kirkwood JM. Temozolomide, a novel alkylating agent with activity in the central nervous system, may improve the treatment of advanced metastatic melanoma. Oncologist. 2000;5(2):144–51.
19. Haubner F, Ohmann E, Pohl F, Strutz J, Gassner HG. Wound healing after radiation therapy: review of the literature. Radiat Oncol. 2012;7:162.

20. Wen PY, Kesari S. Malignant gliomas in adults. N Engl J Med. 2008;359:492–507.
21. Fayers P, Machin D. Quality of life: The assessment, analysis and interpretation of patient-reported outcomes. West Sussex, England: John Wiley & Sons; 2007.
22. Karnofsky DA, Burchenal JH. The clinical evaluation of chemotherapeutic agents in cancer. In: MacLeod CM, editor. Evaluation of chemotherapeutic agents. New York: Columbia University Press; 1949. p. 191–205.
23. Krabbe PFM, Peerenboom L, Langenhoff BS, Ruers TJM. Responsiveness of the generic EQ-5D summary measure compared to the disease-specific EORTC QLQ C-30. Qual Life Res. 2004;13:1247–53.
24. Taphoorn MJ, Claassens L, Aaronson NK, Coens C, Mauer M, Osoba D, et al. An international validation study of the EORTC brain cancer module (EORTC QLQ-BN20) for assessing health-related quality of life and symptoms in brain cancer patients. Eur J Cancer. 2010;46:1033–40.
25. Taphoorn MJ, Stupp R, Coens C, Osoba D, Kortmann R, van den Bent MJ, et al. Health-related quality of life in patients with glioblastoma: a randomised controlled trial. Lancet Oncol. 2005;6:937–44.
26. Kirson ED, Gurvich Z, Schneiderman R, Dekel E, Itzhaki A, et al. Disruption of cancer cell replication by alternating electric fields. Cancer Res. 2004;64:3288–95.
27. Kirson ED, Dbalý V, Tovarys F, Vymazal J, Soustiel JF, Itzhaki A, et al. Alternating electric fields arrest cell proliferation in animal tumor models and human brain tumors. Proc Natl Acad Sci U S A. 2007;104:10152–7.
28. Kanner AA, Wong ET, Villano JL, Ram Z, EF-11 Investigators. Post Hoc analyses of intention-to-treat population in phase III comparison of NovoTTF-100A™ system versus best physician's choice chemotherapy. Semin Oncol. 2014;41 Suppl 6:S25–34.
29. Kaasa S, Bjordal K, Aaronson N, Moum T, Wist E, Hagen S, et al. The EORTC core quality of life questionnaire (QLQ-C30): validity and reliability when analysed with patients treated with palliative radiotherapy. Eur J Cancer. 1995;31A:2260–3.

# Chapter 10
# Future Directions for Tumor Treating Fields

**Eric T. Wong, Minesh P. Mehta, Andrew A. Kanner, and Manmeet S. Ahluwalia**

Future evaluation of the efficacy of Tumor Treating Fields (TTFields) as delivered by the Optune® device will focus upon combination therapies for glioblastoma and monotherapy for other cancer types. Several clinical trials are being conducted and others are being planned for investigating use of TTFields in combination with stereotactic radiosurgery (SRS) and bevacizumab for glioblastoma, and as local treatment for non-small cell lung cancer brain metastasis, systemic lung cancer, mesothelioma, pancreatic cancer, and ovarian cancer. It is noteworthy that the testing of TTFields in humans started in neuro-oncology, initially for the treatment of recurrent glioblastomas (NCT00379470) [1] and later in newly diagnosed glioblastomas (NCT00916409) [2]. This route of development for a new anti-cancer therapy is highly unusual because treatments in neuro-oncology were traditionally adopted

E.T. Wong, M.D. (✉)
Division of Neuro-Oncology, Department of Neurology, Beth Israel Deaconess Medical Center, Boston, MA, USA

Department of Physics, University of Massachusetts in Lowell, Lowell, MA 01854, USA
e-mail: ewong@bidmc.harvard.edu

M.P. Mehta, M.D.
Department of Radiation Oncology, University of Maryland Medical Center, Baltimore, MD, USA
e-mail: mmehta@umm.edu

A.A. Kanner, M.D.
Stereotactic Radiosurgery Unit, Department of Neurosurgery, Tel Aviv Sourasky Medical Center, Tel Aviv University, Tel Aviv, Israel
e-mail: andrewk@tlvmc.gov.il

M.S. Ahluwalia, M.D.
Burkhardt Brain Tumor and Neuro-Oncology Center, Neurological Institute, Cleveland Clinic, Cleveland, OH, USA
e-mail: ahluwam@ccf.org



E.T. Wong (ed.), *Alternating Electric Fields Therapy in Oncology*,
DOI 10.1007/978-3-319-30576-9_10

from established therapies from other disease sites, when the accompanying pre-clinical scientific data on the mechanisms of action have been firmly established. The two pivotal trials conducted in glioblastoma have helped to establish TTFields as a *bona fide* anti-cancer treatment that merits investigation in other types of malignancies outside the central nervous system. In this chapter, we will discuss current and emerging clinical trials that utilize TTFields alone or in combination with other modalities of treatment for glioblastoma and other central nervous system tumors (Table 10.1), and as monotherapy or combination therapy for systemic malignancies (Table 10.2).

## Combination Treatments Using Tumor Treating Fields for Glioblastoma

The rationale for combining TTFields with SRS for recurrent glioblastoma is based on prior SRS trials that demonstrated a survival rate of 8 to 10 months [3–5]. Although not statistically comparable, especially because of significant differences in patient selection, survival after SRS appears favorable when compared to chemotherapy [6, 7]. Furthermore, from a radiobiological standpoint, large fraction radiotherapy might potentiate immune-mediated anti-tumor activity [8, 9]. The addition of TTFields after SRS may further potentiate this effect because tumor cells exposed to alternating electric fields exhibit cell surface expression of calreticulin and the secretion of HMGB1, both of which are required to generate immunogenic cell death [10–12]. In a retrospective analysis of patients with poor prognosis recurrent glioblastoma, the addition of SRS to TTFields therapy prolonged survival when compared to TTFields alone, with a median overall survival of 12 (95 % CI 4–20) months for SRS plus TTFields versus 4 (95 % CI 2–6) months for TTFields alone ($p=0.0036$), recognizing that different patients were selected for these treatment approaches [13]. Taken together, there is a biological rationale underpinning the combination of TTFields and SRS.

Bevacizumab is a humanized monoclonal antibody that inhibits the action of vascular endothelial growth factor and has been approved by the U.S. Food and Drug Administration for recurrent glioblastoma. It is another treatment modality that can be combined with TTFields in an effort to prolong the progression-free survival and/or overall survival of patients with recurrent glioblastoma. To date, clinical trials using single-agent bevacizumab for glioblastoma have not shown an improvement in overall survival but have demonstrated a benefit in progression-free survival [14, 15]. However, a *post hoc* analysis of the phase III EF-11 trial for recurrent glioblastoma revealed that the use of TTFields monotherapy among patients who had progressed on bevacizumab ($n=23$) resulted in an improved median overall survival of 6.0 months compared to those treated with chemotherapy ($n=21$) who had a median overall survival of 3.3 months (hazard ratio = 0.43, 95 % CI, 0.22–0.85) [16]. Recurrent glioblastoma patients present a very difficult therapeutic challenge and an area of unmet need, and it is therefore hoped that the combination of TTFields and bevacizumab can potentially prolong their survival. In addition, the

**Table 10.1** Clinical trials using TTFields in central nervous system malignancies.

| Disease | Phase | Treatment | Endpoint | Status | NCT |
|---|---|---|---|---|---|
| Recurrent GBM | Pilot | TTFields + bevacizumab | PFS | Recruiting | NCT01894061 |
| Recurrent GBM | II | TTFields + Bevacizumab | PFS | Recruiting | NCT02663271 |
| Recurrent GBM | II | TTFields + genomic analysis to identify the genetic signature of response | ORR via RANO | Recruiting | NCT01954576 |
| Recurrent GBM (first recurrence) | II | TTFields + bevacizumab/CCNU | AEs, PFS, OS | Pending | NCT02348255 |
| Recurrent GBM (bevacizumab-naïve) | Pilot | TTFields + bevacizumab + SBRT | AEs | Recruiting | NCT01925573 |
| Recurrent GBM | Pilot | TTFields | Response | Recruiting | NCT02441322 |
| Newly diagnosed unresectable GBM | II | TTFields + bevacizumab + TMZ | AEs | Recruiting | NCT02343549 |
| Recurrent atypical and anaplastic meningioma | Pilot | TTFields | PFS | Recruiting | NCT01892397 |
| COMET: 1-5 NSCLC brain metastases (with controlled systemic disease) | II | TTFields vs. best supportive care | Time to cerebral and distant progression | Recruiting | NCT01755624 |
| METIS: 1-10 NSCLC brain metastases | III | TTFields vs. best supportive care | Time to cerebral progression | Recruiting | NCT02831959 |

*AEs* adverse events, *CCNU* lomustine, *GBM* glioblastoma, *NCT* national clinical trial, *NSCLC* non-small cell lung cancer, *ORR* overall response rate, *OS* overall survival, *PFS* progression-free survival, *RANO* Response Assessment in Neuro-Oncology, *SBRT* stereotactic body radiation therapy, *TTFields* Tumor Treating Fields, *TMZ* temozolomide

**Table 10.2** Clinical trials of TTFields in extracranial solid tumor (non-central nervous system) malignancies.

| Trial | Phase | Treatment | Endpoint | Status | NCT |
|---|---|---|---|---|---|
| PANOVA: Newly diagnosed advanced pancreatic | Open-label pilot | TTFields + gemcitabine with/without nab-paclitaxel | AEs | Completed | NCT01971281 |
| INNOVATE: Recurrent ovarian carcinoma | Open-label pilot | TTFields + weekly paclitaxel | AEs | Completed | NCT02244502 |
| STELLAR: Malignant pleural mesothelioma | II | TTFields + pemetrexed + cisplatin/carboplatin | OS | Recruiting | NCT02397928 |
| LUNAR: Advanced non-small cell lung cancer | III | TTFields + anti-PD1 inhibitor or paclitaxel | OS | Planning | Not available |

*AEs* adverse events, *NCT* national clinical trial, *OS* overall survival, *TTFields* Tumor Treating Fields mechanism of action of TTFields is not limited by normalization of the blood brain barrier due to the use of concomitant bevacizumab as noted earlier. The favorable intracranial safety profile of TTFields and bevacizumab suggests that the combination will probably have an acceptable level of toxicity [16, 17]. There is a planned Radiation Therapy Oncology Group (RTOG) Foundation study on TTFields and bevacizumab in patients with recurrent glioblastoma that have progressed on bevacizumab. The primary endpoint is the overall survival rate at 6 months from registration, while the secondary endpoints include overall survival, progression-free survival, objective response rate, and the frequency of treatment-related adverse events.

There are a number of ongoing investigator-initiated trials combining TTFields and bevacizumab (Table 10.1). Two phase II studies are currently evaluating this combination in patients with recurrent glioblastoma (NCT01894061 and NCT02663271). Another investigator-initiated phase II trial is investigating TTFields therapy combined with bevacizumab and carmustine for the treatment of glioblastoma in first relapse (NCT02348255). A fourth study is evaluating the combination of TTFields with bevacizumab and hypofractionated stereotactic irradiation in bevacizumab-naïve patients with recurrent glioblastoma (NCT01925573); an important goal of this trial is to generate preliminary safety data for the concomitant use of fractionated radiation and TTFields. In addition, a phase II study on patients with newly diagnosed glioblastoma is evaluating the efficacy of combining TTFields with temozolomide and bevacizumab in the adjuvant phase of treatment, after initial radiotherapy with concomitant temozolomide and bevacizumab (NCT02343549). Collectively, these ongoing studies reflect the enthusiasm for multimodality combination therapy using TTFields plus other treatments such as bevacizumab and temozolomide, bevacizumab alone, or bevacizumab and radiosurgery or hypofractionated radiotherapy.

One important study is aimed at addressing the issue of finding genomic signatures that may correlate with the response to TTFields treatment in recurrent glioblastomas (NCT01954576). The subjects in the trial are stratified according to whether they are bevacizumab naïve or refractory, and the primary endpoint is overall response rate according to criteria established by Response Assessment in Neuro-Oncology (RANO) [18]. Another study utilizes high resolution magnetic resonance imaging and spectroscopy sequences, repeated at frequent intervals during TTFields treatment, to evaluate and potentially predict therapeutic response (NCT02441322). Together, these studies may offer important insights into the genomic background associated with radiologic response when patients are treated by TTFields.

## Tumor Treating Fields for Brain Metastasis

TTFields are being investigated for the treatment of brain metastasis from non-small cell lung cancer. Preclinical experiments have demonstrated that multiple human lung cancer cell lines, including H1299 (adenocarcinoma), A549 (adenocarcinoma), HTB-182 (squamous cell carcinoma), and HCC827 (adenocarcinoma with mutated

**Table 10.3** Summary of cell line-specific features in response to TTFields.

| Cell line name | Tissue | Disease | Karyotype[a] | Optimal frequency (kHz) | Doubling time (h) |
|---|---|---|---|---|---|
| A2780 | Ovary | Carcinoma | Modal chromosome number =46 | 200 | 18.7 |
| A549 | Lung | Adenocarcinoma | Hypotriploid, modal chromosome number = 86 in 24 % of cells | 150 | 23.8 |
| AsPC-1 | Pancreas | Adenocarcinoma | Not specified | 150 | 54.0 |
| HeLa | Cervix | Adenocarcinoma | Modal number = 82; range = 70–164 | 150 | 24 |
| MCF-7 | Mammary gland: breast | Adenocarcinoma | Hypertriploidy to hypotetraploidy, modal chromosome number = 82 | 150 | 29.3 |
| MDA-MB-231 | Mammary gland: breast | Adenocarcinoma | Near-triploid, modal number =64 | 150 | 29.1 |
| MSTO-211H | Lung | Biphasic mesothelioma | Modal chromosome number = 72 | 150 | 26.4 |
| NC1-H1299 | Lung | Carcinoma; NSCLC | Not specified | 150 | 23.1 |
| NCI-H2052 | Lung | Stage 4, mesothelioma | Not specified | 200 | 18.9 |
| U-87 MG | Brain | Grade IV glioblastoma: astrocytoma | Hypodiploid, modal chromosome number = 44 in 48 % of cells | 200 | 34.0 |
| U-118 MG | Brain | Grade IV glioblastoma: astrocytoma | Hypodiploid, modal chromosome number = 44 in 48 % of cells | 200 | 18.5 |

From Giladi M. et al. Mitotic Spindle Disruption by Alternating Electric Fields Leads to Improper Chromosome Segregation and Mitotic Catastrophe in Cancer Cells. Scientific Reports. 5, 18046; doi: 10.1038/srep18046 (2015).

[a]According to ATCC and/or NCI SKY/M-FISH and CGH Database

epidermal growth factor receptor [EGFR]), had maximal mitotic disruption at an electric field frequency of 150 kHz (Table 10.3) [19, 20]. There was also an additive effect *in vitro* on tumor cell killing when TTFields were combined with cytotoxic chemotherapies such as premetrexed, cisplatin, and paclitaxel in H1299 and HTB182 cells, as well as targeted therapy such as erlotinib for the EGFR-mutated HCC827 cells [19]. Furthermore, using murine Lewis lung carcinoma cells and KLN205 squamous cell carcinoma cells orthotopically implanted into the left lung of C57BL/6 mice, *in vivo* efficacy was also observed when pemetrexed, paclitaxel, or cisplatin was combined with TTFields [19]. Therefore, there is a strong basis for the application of TTFields in human clinical trials because of its known anti-mitotic mechanisms of action, coupled with the observed robust anti-tumor activities *in vitro* and *in vivo*.

The COMET or EF-21 trial was designed to administer TTFields at a frequency of 150 kHz in a phase II randomized study conducted in Europe for non-small cell lung cancer brain metastasis (NCT01755624). Specifically, this trial enrolls patients with 1 to 5 newly diagnosed brain metastases treated initially with standard-of-care local therapy consisting of either SRS alone or surgery plus SRS, and then followed by randomization to receive TTFields therapy or supportive care. The primary endpoint is time to local or distant intracranial progression. Secondary endpoints include overall survival, 6-month intracranial disease control rate, neurocognitive function, quality of life, progression-free survival, and adverse events. A similar trial that is currently being implemented in the United States is the METIS or EF-25 trial (NCT02831959). The design is similar but METIS allows up to 10 brain metastases treated by local therapy and the analysis will be stratified according to the number of metastases [21].

## Tumor Treating Fields for Atypical and Anaplastic Meningioma

Based on the emerging data on TTFields efficacy for recurrent and newly diagnosed glioblastomas, the Optune® device set at 200 kHz is being applied to other central nervous system tumors such as recurrent grade II atypical and grade III anaplastic meningiomas (NCT1892397). The trial is being conducted at multiple sites in the United States and approximately 21 subjects will be enrolled in the study. The primary outcome measure is progression-free survival and the secondary endpoints are overall survival as well as safety and tolerability.

## Ongoing Studies of Tumor Treating Fields for Extracranial Solid Tumors

The effect of TTFields was also investigated preclinically in AsPC-1 and BxPC-2 human pancreatic adenocarcinoma cell lines, and the reported optimal frequency for anti-mitotic effects is 150 kHz [20, 22]. Interestingly, TTFields caused an increase in cell volume in both AsPC-1 and BxPC-2 cells, a finding consistent with aberrant cytokinesis [20, 23]. These encouraging findings led to PANOVA, a double-arm, nonrandomized, open-label pilot trial, for advanced pancreatic carcinoma testing the safety of add-on TTFields to gemcitabine or to gemcitabine plus nab-paclitaxel (NCT01971281). This trial has completed patient accrual in Europe. Preliminary safety results from 20 enrolled subjects demonstrated 14 (70 %) had serious adverse events, of which 6 (30 %) were hematological, 9 (45 %) were gastrointestinal, and 3 (15 %) were pulmonary events [24]. There was 1 (5 %) fatality from intestinal perforation. Dermatitis, a known side effect of TTFields therapy, was reported in 10 (50 %) subjects and 2 (10 %) were grade 3 in severity but resolved with treatment. Six (30 %) had a partial response and another 6 (30 %) had stable disease. Therefore, the data available thus far indicate that treatment with TTFields in combination with gemcitabine or gemcitabine plus nab-paclitaxel has an acceptable safety profile and warrants further clinical trial investigation.

The optimal TTFields frequency for mitotic disruption is 200 kHz in A2780 ovarian carcinoma cells and *in vitro* experiments have shown a significant decrease in cellular viability and clonogenicity (by 45 % and 24 %, respectively) [20, 25]. *In vivo* mouse studies also showed activity with reduction in tumor luminescence by 40 % and tumor weight by 55 % [25]. These favorable preclinical data led to the development of a pilot phase I/II INNOVATE study of TTFields therapy at 200 kHz given in combination with weekly paclitaxel for recurrent ovarian carcinoma (NCT02244502). The primary endpoints are the adverse event rate and the number of patients prematurely discontinuing TTFields therapy due to skin toxicity. The secondary endpoints include progression-free survival, overall survival, 1-year survival rate, radiological response including duration of response, CA-125 biomarker response rate including response duration, and patient compliance. The study has completed accrual in Europe.

For mesothelioma cells, such as MSTO-211H and NCI-H2052, the optimal frequency for mitotic disruption is 150 kHz and 200 kHz, respectively [20]. Cell viability decreased by about 60 % in both cell lines and clonogenicity decreased by 70 % and 60 %, respectively [20]. A pilot study using the Optune® device at 200 kHz included a patient with pleural mesothelioma who experienced tumor regression near the site of TTFields application and stabilization of other distally located tumors [26]. The phase II STELLAR trial is now testing the efficacy of TTFields in combination with cisplatin or carboplatin for malignant pleural mesothelioma (NCT02397928). The primary endpoint is overall survival, and the secondary endpoints are progression-free survival, response rate, and adverse event rate. This study is being conducted at multiple sites in Europe and is expected to enroll 80 subjects.

Non-small cell lung carcinoma cells, such as H1299 and A549, are disrupted by TTFields at 150 kHz frequency. In particular, A549 cells exhibited marked mitotic spindle disruption upon exposure to TTFields [20]. Based on the preclinical data, the LUNAR or EF-24 trial will be conducted as a randomized study to investigate the benefit of TTFields at the 150 kHz frequency when added to anti-PD1 checkpoint inhibitor therapy or paclitaxel for patients with advanced non-small cell carcinoma of the lung. The primary objective is overall survival and secondary objectives include progression-free survival, radiological response, and quality of life assessment. This study is being planned to enroll subjects in the United States and Europe.

## Conclusions

Future directions for the treatment of glioblastoma by TTFields will involve combination therapies when TTFields are added onto existing regimens or combined with personalized medicine based on genomic profiling. These combinations may include SRS, hypofractionated radiation, bevacizumab, and/or cytotoxic chemotherapy, such as temozolomide or lomustine. Furthermore, a number of trials for the treatment of central nervous system tumors other than glioblastoma have been initiated since 2012, including investigator-initiated trials for recurrent atypical and anaplastic meningiomas. There are ongoing or planned studies for brain metastases from non-small cell lung cancer as well. Lastly, TTFields efficacy is also being studied for the treatment of extracranial solid tumor malignancies, such as pancreatic adenocarcinoma, ovarian carcinoma, pleural mesothelioma, and non-small cell lung carcinoma. As these trial results accumulate over time, TTFields may potentially become an efficacious treatment modality that can be applied to multiple types of malignancies.

## References

1. Stupp R, Wong ET, Kanner AA, Steinberg D, Engelhard H, Heidecke V, et al. NovoTTF-100A versus physician's choice chemotherapy in recurrent glioblastoma: a randomised phase III trial of a novel treatment modality. Eur J Cancer. 2012;48(14):2192–202.
2. Stupp R, Taillibert S, Kanner AA, Kesari S, Steinberg DM, Toms SA, et al. Maintenance therapy with tumor-treating fields plus temozolomide vs temozolomide alone for glioblastoma. A randomized clinical trial. JAMA. 2015;314:2535–43.
3. Fokas E, Wacker U, Gross MW, Henzel M, Encheva E, Engenhart-Cabillic R. Hypofractionated stereotactic reirradiation of recurrent glioblastomas. A beneficial treatment option after high-dose radiotherapy? Strahlenther Onkol. 2009;185:235–40.
4. Hall WA, Djalilian HR, Sperduto PW, Cho KH, Gerbi BJ, Gibbons JP, et al. Stereotactic radiosurgery for recurrent malignant gliomas. J Clin Oncol. 1995;13:1642–8.
5. Shrieve D, Alexander E, Wen PY, Fine HA, Kooy HM, Black PM, et al. Comparison of stereotactic radiosurgery and brachytherapy in the treatment of recurrent glioblastoma multiforme. Neurosurgery. 1995;36:275–84.
6. Wong ET, Hess KR, Gleason MJ, Jaeckle KA, Kyritsis AP, Prados MD, et al. Outcomes and prognostic factors in recurrent glioma patients enrolled onto phase II clinical trials. J Clin Oncol. 1999;17:2572–8.
7. Bokstein F, Blumenthal DT, Corn BW, Gez E, Matceyevsky D, Shtraus N, et al. Stereotactic radiosurgery (SRS) in high-grade glioma: judicious selection of small target volumes improves results. J Neurooncol. 2015;126:551–7.

8. Postow MA, Callahan MK, Barker CA, Yamada Y, Yuan J, Kitano S, et al. Immunologic correlates of the abscopal effect in a patient with melanoma. N Engl J Med. 2012;366:925–31.
9. Dewan MZ, Galloway AE, Kawashima N, Dewyngaert JK, Babb JS, Formenti SC, et al. Fractionated but not single-dose radiotherapy induces an immune-mediated abscopal effect when combined with anti-CTLA-4 antibody. Clin Cancer Res. 2009;15:5379–88.
10. Lee SX, Wong ET, Swanson KD. Disruption of cell division within anaphase by tumor treating electric fields (TTFields) leads to immunogenic cell death. Neuro-Oncology. 2013;15:66–7.
11. Kepp O, Senovilla L, Vitale I, Vacchelli E, Adjemian S, Agostinis P, et al. Consensus guidelines for the detection of immunogenic cell death. Oncoimmunology. 2014;3:e955691.
12. Kepp O, Tesniere A, Schlemmer F, Michaud M, Senovilla L, Zitvogel L, et al. Immunogenic cell death modalities and their impact on cancer treatment. Apoptosis. 2009;14:364–75.
13. Mahadevan A, Barron L, Floyd SR, Kasper E, Wong ET. Survival benefit of tumor treating fields plus stereotactic radiosurgery for recurrent malignant gliomas. J Clin Oncol. 2015;33(Suppl):e13036.
14. Gilbert MR, Dignam JJ, Armstrong TS, Wefel JS, Blumenthal DT, et al. A randomized trial of bevacizumab for newly diagnosed glioblastoma. N Engl J Med. 2014;370:699–708.
15. Chinot OL, Wick W, Mason W, Henriksson R, Saran F, Nishkawa R, et al. Bevacizumab plus radiotherapy-temozolomide for newly diagnosed glioblastoma. N Engl J Med. 2014;370: 709–22.
16. Kanner AA, Wong ET, Villano JL, Ram Z. Post hoc analyses of intention-to-treat population in phase III comparison of NovoTTF-100A™ system versus best physician's choice chemotherapy. Semin Oncol. 2014;41 Suppl 6:S25–34.
17. Zuniga RM, Torcuator R, Jain R, Anderson J, Doyle T, Ellika S, et al. Efficacy, safety and patterns of response and recurrence in patients with recurrent high-grade gliomas treated with bevacizumab plus irinotecan. J Neurooncol. 2009;91:329–36.
18. Wen PY, Macdonald DR, Reardon DA, Cloughesy TF, Sorensen AG, Galanis E, et al. Updated response assessment criteria for high-grade gliomas: Response Assessment in Neuro-Oncology working group. J Clin Oncol. 2010;28:1963–72.
19. Giladi M, Weinberg U, Schneiderman RS, Porat Y, Munster M, Voloshin T, et al. Alternating electric fields (tumor-treating fields therapy) can improve chemotherapy treatment efficacy in non-small cell lung cancer both in vitro and in vivo. Semin Oncol. 2014;41 Suppl 6:S35–41.
20. Giladi M, Schneiderman RS, Voloshin T, Porat Y, Munster M, Blat R, et al. Mitotic spindle disruption by alternating electric fields leads to improper chromosome segregation and mitotic catastrophe in cancer cells. Sci Rep. 2015;5:18046.
21. https://www.novocuretrial.com/metis/.
22. Giladi M, Schneiderman RS, Porat Y, Munster M, Itzhaki A, Mordechovich D, et al. Mitotic disruption and reduced clonogenicity of pancreatic cancer cells in vitro and in vivo by tumor treating fields. Pancreatology. 2014;14:54–63.
23. Gera N, Yang A, Holtzman TS, Lee SX, Wong ET, Swanson KD. Tumor treating fields perturb the localization of septins and cause aberrant mitotic exit. PLoS One. 2015;10:e0125269.
24. Rivera F, Gallego J, Guillen C, Benavides M, Lopez-Martin JA, Betticher DC, et al. PANOVA: a pilot study of TTFields concomitant with gemcitabine for front-line therapy in patients with advanced pancreatic adenocarcinoma. J Clin Oncol. 2016;34(Suppl 4S):269.
25. Munster M, Roberts CP, Schmelz EM, Giladi M, Blat R, Schneiderman RS, et al. Alternating electric fields (TTFields) in combination with paclitaxel are therapeutically effective against cancer cells in vitro and in vivo. Cancer Res 2015;75(15 Suppl):Abstract 5365.
26. Salzberg M, Kirson E, Palti Y, Rochlitz C. Pilot study with very low-intensity, intermediate-frequency electric fields in patients with locally advanced and/or metastatic solid tumors. Onkologie. 2008;31:362–5.

# Index




E.T. Wong (ed.), *Alternating Electric Fields Therapy in Oncology*,
DOI 10.1007/978-3-319-30576-9

Printed in the United States
By Bookmasters